THE WOMEN'S GUIDE TO STRESS RELIEF IN 7 EASY STEPS

Books in the Healthy Home Library Series from St. Martin's Paperbacks

THE WOMEN'S GUIDE TO STRESS RELIEF IN 7 EASY STEPS

Deborah Mitchell

A Lynn Sonberg Book

St. Martin's Paperbacks

Notice: This book is intended as a reference volume only, not as a medical manual. The information given here is designed to help you make informed decisions about your health. It is not intended as a substitute for any treatment that may have been prescribed by your doctor. If you suspect that you have a medical problem, we urge you to seek competent medical help.

Mention of specific companies, organizations, or authorities in this book does not imply endorsement by the author or publisher, nor does mention of specific companies, organizations, or authorities imply that they endorse this book, its author or the publisher.

Internet addresses given in this book were accurate at the time it went to press.

THE WOMEN'S GUIDE TO STRESS RELIEF IN 7 EASY STEPS

Copyright © 2013 by Lynn Sonberg.

All rights reserved.

For information address St. Martin's Press, 175 Fifth Avenue, New York, NY 10010.

EAN: 978-1-250-02629-3

Printed in the United States of America

St. Martin's Paperbacks edition / November 2013

St. Martin's Paperbacks are published by St. Martin's Press, 175 Fifth Avenue, New York, NY 10010.

10 9 8 7 6 5 4 3 2 1

Dedicated to
Antonio Carlos Jobim,
my 4-legged feline
stress reducer

CONTENTS

INTRODUCTION

When I first mentioned to my female friends that I was doing research on a book about women and stress, every one of them, without exception, had a comment that was something similar to (1) "Stress! That's the story of my life!" (accompanied by a sigh, shrug, or a mournful look), or (2) "I wish I knew how to could cope with it better."

This unscientific survey, along with my personal experiences and my then limited knowledge of the scientific literature on the topic of stress, were more than enough to convince me that this book had to include input from two sets of experts: the scientists/researchers who do the legwork and publish their findings about stress, its causes, and how to help manage it; and women who experience and deal with stress on a daily basis.

Researchers have found—and many women would agree—that men and women do not handle or react to stressful situations in the same way. Myrna, for example, is a thirty-five-year-old divorced mother of two girls, six and eight, who gets up at five A.M. every weekday to get her children ready for school, then prepares herself for the thirty-minute drive to the high school where she teaches biology. "By the end of the school day I'm exhausted," she says. "I love what I teach, but the demands of managing teenagers and commanding their attention are mentally and emotionally draining."

Once she leaves school, there are more demands on Myrna's psyche. She picks up the girls at her mother's house, makes dinner, helps with homework, grades papers, pays bills, monitors baths and bedtime, and tumbles into bed, too exhausted to cry or scream, although she feels like doing both.

"At that moment, and for many, many more moments like it every day, I just want to stop and cry or talk to someone, just keep talking and crying until I get it all out. I have female friends who often feel the same way about their lives. Yet when my boyfriend, who is an account executive, gets stressed, he just wants to kick back with a ballgame on TV or play golf instead of talking about it. He deals with stress by zoning out, while I need to let it out."

How do you deal with stress? Do you understand the origins of your stress? Do you know the impact stress can have on your body, mind, and spirit? Do you believe there are ways to effectively and healthfully eliminate, reduce, and manage stress? Are you ready to learn more about these techniques and how other women have incorporated them into their lives?

HOW TO USE THIS BOOK

If you've answered yes to any of those questions, you've come to the right place. Consider this book your resource for managing and banishing stress. First, however, you will need to identify the stressors in your life. Sure, you think you know them all, but you may be surprised at what you're hiding from yourself! Therefore, part of the goal of part 1, Understand Your Stress, is being honest with yourself and about your stress. In these first two chapters, you will learn (1) why women experience so much stress in their lives, (2) how to identify the stressors in your own life, (3) about DROP, a new perspective that can help you eliminate or manage the stress in your life, (4) what perceived stress is and how it affects your health, and (5) about the toll chronic stress can take not only on your mind but on your body and spirit as well.

Then in part 2, Manage (and Banish) Your Stress, you will learn how you and other women can cope with and manage stress in many different ways that will fit into your current lifestyle, perhaps using techniques you never imagined. Before you even start part 2, I will ask you to make a plan using what you already learned in part 1 about identifying and eliminating stress. The plan will incorporate many of the stress-reducing tools explained throughout the seven steps in part 2. Each step also shares stress-reducing plans other women have used to restore balance and sanity to their lives, providing you with ideas you can consider as well.

PART 1

Understand Your Stress

How well do you understand stress? Although stress is something you experience every day to one degree or another, it is much more than a response to situations, people, or other things in your life that keep you feeling tense, frazzled, or on edge.

In fact, the roots of stress go deep, and the results often branch out and impact every corner of your life. Before you can effectively face, manage, and banish the stranglehold stress may have on your physical, mental, emotional, and spiritual well-being, you need to better understand this thing called stress. That's the purpose of part 1.

CHAPTER 1

Why Women Are So Stressed

On the surface, the questions "Why are women so stressed?" or "What causes stress in women?" may seem easy to answer. "My kids and their demands stress me out." "I have too much to do and not enough time to do it!" "I don't know, but I just seem to be crazy busy!" "I can't find the time to relax!" "My life is unmanageable." These are some of the common responses to these questions, but do these comments *really* answer the questions?

Yet often women need to go beneath the surface and dig out the *real* stressors in their lives. This is a critical first step, because you can't work to eliminate or manage the stress-producing or stress-triggering events or circumstances in your life if you don't know what they are. To accurately identify the stressors in your life, you need to be completely honest with yourself and your feelings . . . and this self-examination may not be comfortable at first. But is living with chronic stress comfortable? No! As you probably already know, the first step is the hardest, but I know you can do it!

This chapter has two goals: help you and other women identify why you feel so stressed, and introduce a way to eliminate stress using the DROP approach. (There's a detailed discussion of DROP later in this chapter.) So get ready to understand the anatomy and natural process of stress, to identify the stressors in your life, and how you can start to eliminate and/or manage them in effective, healthful, and enjoyable ways.

WHAT IS STRESS?

We all know what stress is, right? Not having enough time to do everything you need to accomplish, bills you can't afford to pay, sitting in traffic jams, going through a divorce, losing a loved one, having your car break down, losing your job. True, all of these can be stressful situations, but everyone responds to circumstances such as these in a different way or, more precisely, to varying degrees.

Tara, for example, a forty-five-year-old claims adjuster, unexpectedly lost her job during a recent restructuring of her company. Stressful? It could have been, but Tara, who had been thinking seriously about moving from Ohio and applying for several positions in North Carolina near her sister and family said it was the "kick in the butt" she needed. "A week before I lost my job, my sister sent me an e-mail and asked me what it was going to take to get me to make up my mind, that she had several job opportunities for me. Well, losing my job was what it took!"

While I have listed a few examples of stressful situations, they don't answer the question "What is stress?" Stress is a person's response to interactions with external pressures, demands, or stimuli that a person perceives as exceeding her adaptive abilities and that somehow threaten her well-being. Stress is both an external response that scientists can measure (e.g., skin reactions such as sweating or flushing, changes in hormone levels) and an internal reaction that is interpreted emotionally and mentally.

Stress often has a partner in crime called *anxiety,* and although they may have different definitions, the body responds to them in similar ways. While stress is how the body reacts to a real situation, anxiety refers to fear or a general apprehension that something might happen (as in "what if the plane I'm traveling in next week crashes," or becoming anxious over whether it will rain next week when the entire family is coming over for a barbecue).

Stress is a natural part of life, and it has a good gal/bad gal persona. Although stress can be a positive, effective motivator and a creative force, as when you buy a new house and face the challenge of renovating it or you get a promotion that means more money, there is also the dark side of stress. That's the side that includes chronic, persistent stress that can steal away your physical, emotional, and mental health and gnaw away at your spiritual fortitude. The impact of chronic stress on your body, mind, and spirit are discussed in detail in chapter 2.

The secret of living with stress in your life is to roll with, enjoy, and cope with mild and moderate stress and learn how to ward off and/or most effectively eliminate or manage chronic stress. That's what this book can help you do.

THE ANATOMY OF STRESS: TELOMERES

An exciting discovery in the realm of stress and aging is the presence and function of telomeres, which are often referred to as caps or lids located on the ends of chromosomes. Telomeres have several functions, but the primary one is to protect the ends of the chromosomes from damage as cells reproduce. As part of the natural aging process, telomeres gradually become shorter and shorter until the cells can no longer divide and they die. Rather than die, some cells linger on and cause damage to other cells.

Stress, depression, and trauma can speed up the shortening of telomeres, and thus also accelerate the aging process. Other factors that can wear down your telomeres include obesity, lack of physical exercise, and lack of certain nutrients, especially antioxidants.

The encouraging news about telomeres and stress comes from Dr. Elizabeth Blackburn who, along with two colleagues, received the 2009 Nobel Prize in Physiology or Medicine for their discovery of how telomeres protect chromosomes. The year before she received that honor, Blackburn, together with Dr. Dean Ornish, a pioneer in nutritional medicine, president and founder of the nonprofit Preventive Medicine Research Institute in California, and clinical professor of medicine at the University of California, San Francisco, reported in *The Lancet Oncology* that "lifestyle changes can significantly increase telomerase [an enzyme that increases telomere length] activity and consequently telomere maintenance capacity in human immune-system cells."

The implications of the research and findings concerning telomeres and stress are life-changing. Basically, stressful situations and events trigger a response, but it is up to you how you respond and manage the stress that may accompany that response. You have the choice to modify how you respond by utilizing stress management tools—many examples of which are presented in Part 2 of this book—to significantly reduce or eliminate the effects of stress in your life. When you use those tools, you take control of your physical, mental, emotional, and spiritual health and well-being.

According to Dr. Blackburn, "Telomeres are the only

part of the genome [the complete set of genetic material of an organism] itself that can be changed by lifestyle choices, and hence telomere length measurements can provide valuable feedback on one's disease risks." The choice is up to you.

Telomeres are such an important part of stress and how it affects the body, I refer to them throughout the book, and in fact return to them again in chapter 2, so stay tuned!

HORMONES AND STRESS

Your boss is on the rampage. Your kids are fighting over who gets to use the computer—again. You're stuck in traffic and you're late for an appointment. Any of these situations may cause your muscles to tighten, your stomach to churn, or make you feel like you want to shout a few choice words. But what's happening on a hormonal level? Plenty.

In fact, one of the reasons why women and men don't react to stressful situations in the same way has to do with hormones, and there are three of them we need to discuss: cortisol, epinephrine, and oxytocin.

Let's say you're in a traffic jam and you're already late for a presentation you are supposed to give for your company. You're on your cell phone (hands-free, of course, because you don't need the added stress of getting caught talking on the phone while driving) explaining to your secretary that you're running late because of traffic. People around you are honking their horns. (Where do they think you can go?) You want to block them out but you're not having too much success.

Internally, your hormones are reacting to the traffic and honking as well. Both cortisol and epinephrine step up and cause your blood glucose (sugar) and blood pressure to rise. Cortisol provides an extra feature: it suppresses your immune system, making it less effective at fighting the bad guys.

Up to this point, hormones in both men and women would activate in the same ways in response to a traffic jam or other stressful situation. But then things change. The third hormone, oxytocin, enters the picture after cortisol and epinephrine have made their way into the bloodstream, and in women oxytocin, which is released from the brain, puts some braking moves on both cortisol and epinephrine production. Oxytocin is a "love" hormone, which means it promotes feelings of calm, nurturing, and relaxation.

Men, however, secrete much smaller amounts of oxytocin, hence they have a tendency to react to stress by either suppressing the stress reaction deep inside themselves or fighting back—the old "fight-or-flight response." Also known as the acute stress response, the fight-or-flight response refers to a physical reaction individuals have when something physically or mentally terrifying or stressful occurs. This response was first described in the 1920s by physiologist Walter Cannon, who noted that people experience a series of rapidly occurring chemical reactions when they are faced with a threat.

"Tend and Befriend"

In a groundbreaking study on stress in women and men published in 2000, an entirely new light was cast on the subject. The researchers from the University of California, Los Angeles, (UCLA) explained that while the traditional fight-or-flight view of stress may represent the main physical responses males and females have to stressful situations, they proposed that females are more apt to respond with a pattern they called "tend-and-befriend."

That is, women generally react to stress by engaging in nurturing (tending) activities such as caregiving to protect themselves and others, as well as reaching out (befriending) to friends and others to help them deal with the stress. According to the researchers, the biology that lies at the core of the tend-and-befriend pattern suggests oxytocin plus the female sex hormones are involved in the stress response. Since men release much less oxytocin, they tend to respond more frequently with a fight-or-flight reaction.

WHAT'S SPECIAL ABOUT WOMEN'S STRESS?

If you read the previous section on men, women, stress, and hormones, you already know that one thing special about women's stress involves hormones. But it goes deeper than that. The presence and activity of those hormones directly impact how women respond to stressful situations. Psychologist Carl E. Pickhardt, PhD, who has authored dozens of books on various aspects of parenting (and parenting is one of the main sources of chronic stress for women), has pointed out that the greatest stressor for women is usually associated with a relationship: that is, there is trouble with, or the loss or failure of, a relationship, whether it be with a parent, friend, child, or partner.

Women tend to work hard at "keeping it together," maintaining the solidarity and harmony in relationships. They also tend to be self-sacrificing and to act as caregivers— paying attention to and nurturing children, parents, partners, and friends, often at the risk of not tending to their own needs. All of these efforts can take a significant toll on a woman's physical, emotional, mental, and spiritual health unless she takes steps to curtail or stop it.

For men, the greatest stressor is usually performance failure, especially concerning a job or career, sexual prowess, and failure in sports or any type of competition. That's not to say women don't experience stress related to their careers or that they are not competitive, but simply the core energy feeding a woman's stress tends to be different from a man's.

BAD NEWS AND STRESS

One doesn't have to look far to find bad news: whether you get your news from the Internet, the TV, radio, print media, or your family and friends, disturbing, often horrifying news is everywhere. And where there's bad news, women tend to react to it differently than men. That was the finding of a 2012 study by Sonia Lupien and her team from the University of Montreal, although your own experiences probably already have led you to the same conclusion.

Lupien exposed groups of men and women to two types of news: neutral and negative. After everyone had read a series of headlines in their assigned categories, they underwent standard psychological stress tests. Women who had been exposed to negative headlines had higher levels of cortisol after the test when compared with men and with women who had read the neutral headlines. In addition, the day after the study the women who read negative headlines had a greater chance of remembering and reliving the emotions they felt than the men did. This is another example of how women hold on to and internalize their stress while men tend to let it go.

IDENTIFYING THE REAL CAUSES OF STRESS

Now that we've dissected stress, let's see if you can identify the real causes of the stress in your life. We're probably all familiar with the pat answers to what causes stress in a woman's life: children, husband/partner, job, parents, money problems, getting older, never having enough time.

Although these are all legitimate answers, they don't go deep enough. If you can pinpoint exactly what it is about your job that is stressful, for example, then you can take the appropriate action. Until you do, any efforts you make at reducing, eliminating, or managing your stress may actually result in your experiencing more tension and anxiety as you realize you are not accomplishing your goal.

That means it's time to do some soul-searching, and when you do, you may discover that it's not really your job, per se, that is the stressor, but something else. For example, you might ask yourself the following questions:

✓ Is there something specific about the work you do that is stressful? That is, is there a particular task or aspect of your job that causes you great anxiety? Is there more than one task that causes you to feel stressed? Is it possible that you are just not suited for the work you do, and that you need to find another job?

✓ Do you have a stressful relationship with one or more of your co-workers? What specifically about that person (or persons) causes you stress, anxiety, or to feel uncomfortable?

✓ Is your relationship with your boss causing your stress? What specifically about your relationship or your boss is at the root of your tension or discomfort?

✓ Is your commute to work so stressful it has a negative impact on the rest of your day?

✓ Are you stressed at work because of the environment (e.g., lighting, odors, feeling confined)?

You can easily modify these questions to apply to other stressful situations in your life. For example: "Is your relationship with————causing your stress?" or "Are you stressed (at the gym, volunteering at the church, at home, or other) because of the environment?" And so on.

Roseanne is a marketing account manager who said she found her job to be very stressful. "The worst part of my day is the morning, and especially the days I have meetings before noon, which happens several times a week. I'm typically prepared for these meetings, yet I still feel really tense and unsettled, and I'm not really sure why."

When Roseanne took some time to more closely examine her dilemma, she discovered that it wasn't the meetings or her job that was stressing her out, but the commute to work. She had a fifty- to sixty-minute drive on packed freeways and city streets every morning, and by the time she arrived, her nerves were on edge. When she thought more clearly about her drive to work, she admitted that it left her feeling tense for hours, and that she didn't quite feel herself until about noon. Another factor she had not thought about was that she really enjoyed having a cup of green tea in the morning because she said it relaxed her. However, because she was afraid she would need a bathroom break while going to work, she skipped morning tea during the week.

Once Roseanne identified the root of her stress, she was able to take steps that effectively addressed it. Since she was not able to find an alternative to driving to work (but she did manage to arrange to work at home several days a month!), Roseanne came up with a solution: she practices guided meditation for ten minutes before leaving for work, plays soothing music in her car's CD player, and then spends ten minutes in quiet meditation after she arrives at her office. And she treats herself to that much-needed cup of green tea.

"I even put a sign on my door, MEDITATING—DO NOT KNOCK OR DISTURB, and it works," said Roseanne. "A few other people in the office have started doing the same thing. I never realized I was a trendsetter! But the biggest benefit is that I feel so much better, less stressed. The combination of guided meditation and the soothing music has made a big difference, plus the mere fact that I discovered the reason for my anxiety and took positive action to correct it." For those without a private office, a quiet corner in a lunch area or outside may serve the same purpose.

If you can identify the real roots of your stress, then you can take effective steps to eliminate or reduce it (using the DROP approach, discussed below) and/or manage it, which is explored in step 2 of this book. If, however, you are stressed out and can't clearly identify the reason, then your chances of relieving your stress are not great. As one woman put it, "If you blow up at your partner because he put an empty carton of orange juice back in the refrigerator, is the real reason you're stressed and angry because of the empty carton? More than likely his action is just the proverbial straw that broke the camel's back. It's time to find the core reason for your feelings."

Identifying the roots of your stress also can help you see the situation in a new light, with different eyes if you will, so you can then take the most appropriate action. That's what happened for Roseanne, and it can happen for you, too. And one way to take action is to try the DROP approach.

"CRAZY BUSY"

Okay, it's time to be honest with yourself. Are you among the group of people who secretly view stress and being "crazy busy" as a badge of honor? A blog article in the *New York Times* by Tim Kreider entitled "The 'Busy' Trap" explained that "if you live in America in the 21st century you've probably had to listen to a lot of people tell you how busy they are. It's become the default response when you ask anyone how they're doing: 'Busy!' 'So busy.' 'Crazy busy.' It is, pretty obviously, a boast disguised as a complaint. And the stock response is a kind of congratulation: 'That's a good problem to have,' or 'Better than the opposite.'"

Did you just see yourself in that paragraph? Do you feel guilty if you aren't going somewhere or doing something productive all the time? Are you among those who are busy all the time, as Kreider noted, "because they're addicted to busyness and dread what they might have to face in its absence"? If you have answered yes to any of these questions, congratulations for being honest.

Here's another question for you: If you have children, are you doing the same thing with them, scheduling their time or making sure they have their calendar so full of activities and events they don't have time to be kids, to relax, to use their imagination?

Now, it's up to you. Do you sincerely want to change and reconnect—or possibly connect for the first time—with yourself, your family and friends, and your world? You have the power to take back control of your life and to banish and manage the stress in your life. Is it really healthy physically, mentally, emotionally, or spiritually to be so busy all the time? Or is it just crazy?

ELIMINATING STRESSORS: THE DROP APPROACH

It's one thing to identify the stressors in your life, and you can congratulate yourself for recognizing them. You should also give yourself a pat on the back as you move ahead in this book and learn more about how to manage stress in effective, healthful ways. However, it's easier and healthier to prevent disease (and similarly, chronic stress and all its health consequences) than to treat it. That's why it's critical to learn how to eliminate stress.

At the same time, let's remember that stress is a part of life. New stressors will keep coming into your life and you will need to face them. However, if you are forearmed with the right tools then you will be better equipped to take stressors in stride, or at least with a minimum of collateral damage!

The DROP Approach

Do you believe you deserve a rich, fulfilling life? Do you think stressors in your life are preventing you from realizing that goal? Do you believe you can take charge of your life and eliminate some of its stressors?

If you answer yes to these questions, then you are ready to celebrate your life as a woman, wife/partner, mother/daughter, friend/companion, worker/volunteer, and citizen of the world. You deserve a life that is rich and full, as unencumbered with unnecessary stress as possible. This is not a selfish desire; in fact, eliminating stressors from your life allows you not only to be a more fulfilled person, but to have opportunities to share your richness and joys with others.

The Four Elements of DROP

DROP is an acronym for four different ways to help eliminate stressors. Let's look at each one of these approaches separately.

Delegate

If you're a person who likes to have control over every situation in your life, delegating responsibility to others may be a challenge, but bear with me for a few moments and you will hopefully realize the importance and power of this element of DROP. The ability to delegate tasks to others is an important tool to use because it can allow you to get off the "I gotta" train and let you be the station manager instead of the conductor, coal shoveler, and ticket collector all in one.

Think about a stressful situation or circumstance in your life. Is there someone else who can relieve some of that burden by performing one or more tasks that are now a source of anxiety or stress for you? Can you delegate responsibility to another person at work, school, home, church, or social committee? Or are you caught up in the "I gotta do this" and "I gotta do that" way of thinking, when in reality what you "gotta do" is be willing and able to delegate some of the responsibility elsewhere.

Here are a few suggestions:

- When delegating responsibilities to others, be sure to explain what needs to be done and provide instructions (especially for children or uninitiated spouses/partners) in a gentle and precise way. After all, the goal is to reduce your stress level, not raise it, so it's in your best interests to help ensure the tasks are done correctly.

- Pick one or two tasks around the house that cause you stress and which could be done by another family member and delegate that job to them. It may be walking the dog, cleaning out the litter box, loading the dishwasher, removing the laundry from the dryer and folding it, or vacuuming the living room. You might then take advantage of a few extra moments to relax with guided imagery, yoga, or meditation (see chapters 4 and 5).

- If you are part of a committee at work, church, or in a social group, be sure you know what your responsibilities are and don't volunteer to do more when you know you don't have the time. It's okay to say no when a request or someone else's expectations of you will cause you additional anxiety or stress.

Reduce

Less is more in many cases, and if you can reduce some elements of a stressful situation, you can get more out of life or make your day more pleasant. For example, one woman told me she avoided calling her daughter during the week because she had a way of upsetting her mother with her complaints. "I've learned from experience that talking to my daughter during the week, especially early in the morning, causes me so much stress at work, it affects my ability to do my job. I wait for the weekends when I can decompress."

Do you have similar situations in your life where you can reduce the impact a stressor has on your health? It can be a simple step, such as avoiding particular stores when you know they are crowded if crowds make you tense. A significant tool in the Reduce category is the word "no." In fact, utilizing the word "no" may be the best way for you to reduce stress in your life. Does playing tennis with your neighbor make you extremely tense? Then it's time to say no, and perhaps find something relaxing you can do together. You can begin to reduce stress by implementing effective management and coping skills, such as those discussed in steps 1 through 7.

One area of significant stress can be so-called time-saving or labor-saving devices. Consider whether they are really providing you a service or their presence in your life should be reduced. For example, cell phones and computers have become commonplace and often necessary, but do you really need every latest gadget or all the bells and whistles? Have you come to depend so much on these devices that if one malfunctions or is lost, you are lost as well? Before you buy any new equipment, evaluate whether it will really be useful or end up as a source of unnecessary stress; your evaluation should include the cost of purchasing the device as well as getting it repaired or replaced.

Another factor to remember in the Reduce category is multitasking. Do you really need to cook dinner, talk on your cell phone, and watch your kids all at the same time? You may be familiar with the studies showing that texting while driving or texting while walking is dangerous. Multitasking is a stressful (and potentially hazardous) situation. Try doing one thing at a time, as much as possible. If you are taking a walk, enjoy your surroundings and relax. Reduce your tasks and don't overload your circuits! It's even okay to not do anything once in a while—just take a few moments to be present, meditate, do deep breathing exercises, and be quiet (see chapter 5).

Organize

One of the most important ways to eliminate stress in your life is to practice good organizational skills, which includes organizing your time as well as your environment. People who are organized tend not to waste time looking for things or information: they have ready access. Many women discover that if they stop and think about it, the disorganization in their lives is a significant cause of stress. Once they begin to take stock and make changes, they discover they *do* have more time to get things done, and as a result some of the tension and stress is lifted from their lives.

One simple step you can take is to sit at your computer or take out paper and pen and write down how you spend your time each day. Are the events and tasks in your day organized in a way that is as stress-free as possible?

Some other examples include:

- Are your files organized in a way that allows you to find information easily? Or do you have duplicate files (e.g., five files marked "Car insurance" all filed in different places), stacks of items to be filed, or a catch-all file that desperately needs to be sorted?

- Is your work space, including your desk, computer, calendar, books, and any files, arranged in a way that allows you to be as efficient as possible?

- Do you know what's in your pantry and kitchen cabinets? When it's time to go grocery shopping or prepare a recipe, are your food items arranged in such a way that you know what you have and what you need to buy?

- When you have many errands to run, do you organize them in a way that maximizes your time? For example, you may have six stops to make in one day, and you could write them down or mentally organize them and the routes you will take to complete them so you make the most efficient use of your time.

- Are items in your house organized in ways that make finding them easy and thus not stressful? Are there central locations for important or often-used items such as keys to the cars and other things that require a key, cleaning supplies, batteries, lightbulbs, and medications? Hint: you might want to delegate the responsibility for establishing such locations or organizing them to your children or partner!

Prioritize

What are the most important things you need to do each day? Will the world stop turning if you don't pick up the dry cleaning or vacuum the living room, remember to buy coffee at the supermarket, or clean the bathtub on a particular day? Do you find yourself making promises to do things for others when you know (in the back of your mind) that you don't really have the time to do them but you don't say no? Again, the simple two-letter word "no" is all-important. Ask yourself: "Is this activity, task, or event a priority?" If not, then it may be time for you to say no, or at least put the activity on hold. If you take a moment to prioritize the demands and tasks in your life, then you can eliminate or at least reduce your stress.

You can use one or more of the DROP concepts to help you achieve your goal. Here are a few examples of how other women have used DROP.

Leslie

Leslie, a forty-one-year-old mother of three, found it necessary to return to work full-time as a nurse's assistant when finances got tight and her husband was forced to take a pay cut. When Leslie analyzed her life circumstances, she identified several stressors that were taking a toll: (1) worries about finances, (2) her husband's anxiety about making less money (and feeling like "less of a man"), (3) her feelings of guilt because she wasn't able to spend as much quality time with her children, and (4) her inability to maintain her household as she had done before returning to work. On the positive side, she really enjoyed her job and working with patients.

As Leslie did an honest assessment of her needs, she decided her priority was to take steps to feel better about herself. "I know that sounds selfish," she said, "and I didn't even like to admit it, but I also know myself well enough to realize that if I feel good about what I'm accomplishing, then I am better able to tackle other challenging areas of my life." Leslie gets a sense of accomplishment when her household is running efficiently, but her job was making that goal impossible. She also knew that she liked to maintain as much control as possible over how things were done around the house.

So she utilized another part of the DROP approach. Leslie drew up a chart that delegated household chores and responsibilities among her children (ages six, nine, and ten), her husband, and herself. Each child is responsible for keeping his or her room neat and putting dirty clothes in the laundry room. Everyone shares responsibility for feeding, combing, and cleaning up after the cat on a rotating weekly schedule. Leslie still does most of the cooking, but her husband prepares and cleans up after two meals per week. Everyone has been shown how to properly load the dishwasher, although only Leslie and her husband can turn it on.

Leslie has even adapted some of the chores so that she can spend more time with her children. "Sorting and folding laundry is a 'mommy and kids' activity," she says. "Some gardening chores are also family time, like raking leaves or weeding the garden."

Gayle

"I know I have terrible time-management skills," complains Gayle, a fifty-one-year-old full-time advertising account executive who also is a licensed massage therapist. "I really try to manage my time and steal a few moments for myself to decompress from the stress in my life, but it just seems like time gets away from me. When I have a day off, I make plans to accomplish certain tasks, and then something happens and I don't get them done.

The thing is, I know what I should do—meditate, prioritize, relax—and I just don't do it."

Gayle was experiencing physical symptoms of chronic stress, including daily headaches and stomach upset several times a week, and then she came down with the flu and became too ill to drag herself out of bed. Looking back at the situation, she realizes it was the best thing that could have happened to her.

"The flu knocked me out, and I was forced to stay in bed for nearly a week. So I had plenty of time to review what I was doing with my life, to assess and set my priorities, and come up with a better way to manage my work and my home life. I decided to practice a new word more often—'no'—and even made my first big 'no' decision while I was still stuck in bed. I had been asked to serve on a committee for a local social group, and I knew I didn't want to do it but hadn't had the courage to say no until then. I felt relieved after I made that call!"

To enjoy a balanced, healthful life, it's important to live with stress that keeps you motivated and excited about life while also learning how to manage, cope with, reduce, or eliminate stress that has the potential to be or is harmful. That is your challenge. But before you dive into ways to use the concepts of DROP in your life, let's look at what stress can do to you.

CHAPTER 2

What Stress Does to You

Stress is not a benign event; even though a stressor may be something that happens "out there," such as a family member getting sick or the car breaking down, the shock waves of the stressor hit home: you. And those shock waves can take a tremendous toll on your physical, emotional, mental, and spiritual health. Both stress and its cohort anxiety can manifest in scores of ways and trigger a cascade of health problems and accelerate aging. I am reminded of a woman I met at a dinner for a colleague. I was among a group of six women who were hovering near the appetizer table, nursing red wine and chatting among ourselves. All of us appeared to be in our prime years—fiftyish or so, with a young grandmother among us—but later as we wandered off to our table, one of the women, Vicky, disappeared, and I asked one of the other women, Naomi, where she had gone.

"Oh, Vicky had to call her babysitter. Her two-year-old has a cold, and she wants to check on her." I made a casual remark about her having a baby late in life, and Naomi laughed. "Late? Vicky is thirty-one and has four kids all younger than ten. But I know what you mean. She looks much older, and I'm not surprised. She works two part-time jobs, her husband travels for work most of the time, and Vicky helps take care of her mother, who had a stroke last year. The poor thing is a nervous wreck. I'm surprised she even made it here tonight."

What impact is stress having on your body, mind, and spirit? The goal of this chapter is to assist you in answering that question. By the end, you will hopefully better understand the impact stress can have on your life and know how to identify some of the effects you may have ignored or disregarded and thus open the door to ways to deal with them, which is covered in detail in future chapters.

STRESS AND DOCTORS:
WHAT THEY DON'T TELL YOU

Even though stress is usually a factor in 60 to 80 percent of the visits people make to their primary care doctor, only 3 percent of patients ever get any type of stress management counseling or advice from their health-care providers, according to a study from Beth Israel Deaconess Medical Center (BIDMC) that appeared in the November 19, 2012, issue of the *Archives of Internal Medicine*. In fact, the study's lead author, Aditi Nerurkar, MD, MPH, who is the assistant medical director of BIDMC's Cheng & Tsui Center for Integrative Care, noted that "stress is the elephant in the room. Everyone knows it's there, but physicians rarely talk to patients about it." Why?

Well, stress! The research team evaluated data from more than 34,000 office visits and 1,263 doctors, searching for evidence of doctors who provided their patients with stress management assistance, such as counseling at the visit, offering information on how to reduce stress, and referrals to other professionals to help with stress management.

However, they found a mere 3 percent of doctors offered any type of stress management help, and a big reason for that is stress itself. Gloria Yeh, MD, MPH, director of the Integrative Medicine Fellowship Program at Harvard Medical School and BIDMC, explained that "we know that primary care physicians are overburdened . . . there simply may not be enough time to provide stress management counseling during the office visit."

So what does this mean for you? Don't count on others, not even the medical community, to help you fight stress. It's time to take stress management and stress elimination into your own hands. If you can find a health-care provider who will help you, great! But be prepared to take control of your stress and your life, starting now.

STRESS MAKES IT WORSE

The presence of chronic stress makes physical, emotional, mental, and spiritual problems worse. If you are experiencing a disturbing amount of stress in your life right now, you know what I mean. It's as if you're living on the edge or as if the volume of life is just a bit too loud. Just the mere fact that your muscles tense up when you are stressed can make numerous conditions worse, ranging from headache to back pain, arthritis, fibromyalgia, stomach cramps, menopausal symptoms, and constipation, among others.

Beyond making your muscle tense, chronic stress has other effects on your internal structures. For example, the stress hormone cortisol (introduced in chapter 1) causes the thymus gland to shrink. The thymus plays a key role in regulating the immune system, including the production of white blood cells and their function. Prolonged chronic stress can cause the immune system cells to attack the body, which leads to autoimmune disease such as asthma, allergies, lupus, rheumatoid arthritis, and many others.

Stress also interferes with the production and function of natural killer cells, which are responsible for finding and killing cancer and virus cells. Chronic stress can even speed up the growth of cancer cells. Elevated levels of cortisol also affect the production of brain chemicals called serotonin and dopamine, which are involved in regulating mood.

Here are some disturbing and overwhelming statistics. (1) Every week, about 112 million people take some type of medication that is supposed to relieve stress-related symptoms (see step 7); and (2) between 75 and 90 percent of all visits made to primary care doctors are related to stress. Among the symptoms and conditions related to stress are the following:

Anxiety
Backache
Chronic fatigue
Colds and flu
Depression
Diabetes
Excessive sweating
Fibromyalgia
Gallstones
Gastrointestinal disorders (e.g., Crohn's disease, ulcerative colitis, ulcers)
Hair loss
Headache/migraine
Heart disease
High blood pressure
Immune system disorders
Insomnia
Lack of libido (sex drive)

Memory loss
Mood swings
Muscle tension
Panic attacks
Rapid heartbeat
Skin irritation and rash
Stomach pains
Urinary tract infections
Urinary tract symptoms (e.g., frequent and/or urgent urination)
Weight loss or gain (unexplained)

Scientists have shown that stress can heighten a person's perception of pain and their depth of depression. One of the best examples of this phenomenon has been found in connection with fibromyalgia, a chronic pain condition that primarily affects women and is characterized by depression, fatigue, insomnia, and other life-altering symptoms. Experts believe chronic stress is a trigger for typical fibromyalgia symptoms and have conducted studies to illustrate this point.

In one such study, women with fibromyalgia were matched with healthy women (controls), and all the participants took part in a number of tests for depression, stress, health assessment, and pain. The incidence of depressive symptoms was higher (75 percent) in the women with fibromyalgia than in the controls (25 percent), and there was a clear correlation between symptoms of depression and perceived stress, pain, and the impact on the women's quality of life.

Scientists at Penn State reported on the effects of stress in a National Institutes of Health study published in November 2012. Their findings supported the idea that contrary to popular thought, it's not the stressors in our lives that cause health problems, but how we react to them.

David Almeida, professor of human development and family studies and one of the study's authors, explained that "our research shows that how you react to what happens in your life predicts your chronic health conditions 10 years in the future, independent of your current health and your future stress."

That sounds ominous, doesn't it? Almeida went on to explain that "if you have a lot of work to do today and you are really grumpy because of it, then you are more likely to suffer negative health consequences 10 years from now than someone who also has a lot of work to do today, but doesn't let it bother her." The researchers based their conclusions not only on observations but on cortisol levels collected both in 1995 and in 2005. In addition, they evaluated daily stressors and found that people who were negatively affected by daily stressors and dwelled on them were more likely to experience chronic health problems, especially pain, arthritis, and cardiovascular problems a full decade later.

This information is great food for thought—and action. As you can see, stress has no mercy: it reaches into every cell, tissue, organ, and system in your body, and it also spans time. Stress can both cause and exacerbate symptoms and health problems. However, always keep in mind that once you identify the stressors in your life, you can use DROP and incorporate ways to manage stress utilizing some of the stress reduction tips presented in step 2 or from other sources and significantly improve your health and well-being.

WHAT'S YOUR STRESS THRESHOLD?

The impact of stress on your physical, emotional, mental, and spiritual health depends in large part on your stress threshold. How can you determine your stress threshold? Experts have identified factors that are considered to have a role in how well you can handle stress. Here are some of those factors. How well do you think you rate on each one?

- Your ability to deal with emotions (e.g., do you experience wide mood swings? Do you tend to overreact emotionally, such as crying for no apparent reason or laughing much too loudly or long in a stressful situation?)

- How well you are prepared for stressful events in your life (e.g., do you often feel a sense of panic or doom when thinking about stressful situations? Do you worry excessively about stressful situations, such as losing your job, your children's health, your finances, caring for your parents?)

- The presence of a support network (e.g., do you have a support system that includes family, friends, neighbors, and/or people from your church or other social institution that you can turn to for emotional and/or spiritual support? Do you feel confident about those in your support network?)

- The state of your physical health (e.g., do you have a healthy diet? Do you smoke? Do you exercise regularly?)

- Attitude (e.g., do you generally maintain a positive or negative attitude? How do you think your friends would define your attitude?)

- Your ability to sleep (e.g., do you get enough sleep so that you feel rested? Is your sleep bothered by stress? Do you suffer with insomnia?)

- Sense of control (e.g., do you feel like you have some control over events and stress in your life? Do you often feel hopeless or helpless?)

Now, here are some factors that indicate you are not dealing well with the stress in your life; that is, you have a low stress threshold. For example, do you display any of the following characteristics:

- Chronic headache and/or stomachache

- Restlessness and/or jumpiness

- Problems at work

- Problems with your intimate relationships

- Eating changes (e.g., eating more or eating less, emotional eating [often referred to as mindless eating, which typically leads to weight gain])

- Feeling irritable or short-tempered

- Problems with concentration and/or memory

- Feelings of panic, helplessness, and/or hopelessness

- Loss of a normally healthy sex drive

- Thoughts of harming yourself or suicide

- Increase in the use of tobacco, alcohol, or other drugs

If you are experiencing any of these traits, then chances are your stress threshold is challenged. The more traits you have, the more challenged your stress threshold. But that's okay: identifying and acknowledging your stress threshold is important *if* you use that information to move forward and do something about it, such as working to eliminate and manage your stressors before they manage you.

HEART DISEASE AND STRESS

Heart disease is the number one killer of women in the United States, and is the cause of death in 25 percent of women. Stress is among the risk factors for heart disease, and it also has an impact on others. For example, stress can contribute to the narrowing of blood vessels, which can lead to a rise in blood pressure and the risk for a heart attack. Getting angry can trigger a heart attack, and being depressed increases the risk of developing coronary heart disease by two- to threefold. Depression is twice as common in women as in men. Stress can also cause individuals to engage in unhealthy activities, such as smoking, drinking excess alcohol, eating unhealthy foods, and not exercising, all of which are risk factors for heart disease.

Women also have a few other factors not in their favor when it comes to heart disease. While men and women share many of the same risk factors for heart problems, women who have diabetes are at greater risk than men for coronary heart disease, and use of birth control pills and the onset of menopause also have a negative impact on women's heart-disease risk.

Since heart disease is such a significant health problem among women, it's important to consider the impact of stress on heart function. One side of stress that plays a significant role in heart disease is perceived stress. What is perceived stress? It has been defined as "the general perception that environmental demands exceed perceived capacity regardless of the source of the environmental demand." In other words, if you believe a situation is stressful, then for you it is, even if others do not believe the same or tell you "you shouldn't get upset or stressed over that" or "it's not a big deal." What's important to remember, however, is that you *can* take steps to effectively deal with perceived stress, and one of the first steps you can take is recognizing it (see "The Perceived Stress Scale").

In a study published in December 2012 in the *American Journal of Cardiology,* New York researchers reported on the results of a meta-analysis, which included data from six studies (118,696 total participants). They noted that people who had high levels of perceived stress were 27 percent more likely to develop coronary heart disease compared with individuals who had low perceived stress. The researchers equated the magnitude of high perceived stress with smoking five more cigarettes daily, a 50 mg/dl rise in bad (LDL) cholesterol, or a 2.7/1.4 mmHg increase in blood pressure, all risk factors for heart disease.

The Perceived Stress Scale

The Perceived Stress Scale (PSS) is the most commonly used tool mental health professionals turn to for measuring a person's perception of stress. The scale consists of ten general questions about a person's thoughts and feelings during the last month on routine or everyday situations. An adaptation of the PSS is provided here so you can get an overall idea of how stressful you find different situations in your life to be. Generally, the higher you rate yourself on the negative questions and the lower you score on the positive questions, the greater your level of perceived stress. If you are interested in learning more about the PSS and having a professional work with you on your PSS score, then you should seek the assistance of a mental health provider (see step 7).

PERCEIVED STRESS SCALE

Score each item from 0 to 4. The first six items are negative factors and the next four are positive factors.

0 = never 1 = almost never 2 = sometimes 3 = fairly often 4 = often

During the last month, how often did you feel:

- Like you could not control important aspects in your life

- Extremely upset because an unexpected event or situation occurred

- Stressed out and nervous

- Like you could not cope with all the errands and other things you needed to do

- Angry because of events or situations that occurred outside of your control

- Overwhelmed because events or situations were accumulating beyond your ability to overcome them

- Confident that you were able to handle your personal issues

- That things in your life were going in a positive direction

- Like you were on top of situations in your life

- Like you were in control of irritations in your life

STRESS, TELOMERES, AND YOUR HEALTH

It's another Monday morning, and you're up at the crack of dawn to get the kids ready for school before you race into the shower to prepare yourself for another day at the office. The minute you reach your desk the phone is ringing, your secretary is waiting with papers in her hand, and your calendar for the week is full. Yes, just another hectic, stress-filled Monday morning, to be followed by four more workdays of the same.

According to a 2012 study published in the peer-reviewed medical journal *PLoS ONE,* stress on the job has a negative impact on telomeres (see chapter 1), those tiny "caps" on the ends of chromosomes that protect genetic coding from damage, help cells divide, and play a role in aging and cancer. The Finnish scientists found that individuals who experienced high levels of stress at work were more likely to have short telomeres.

Stress, along with age, exposure to chemicals, and oxidation (free-radical damage) cause telomeres to become shorter. When telomeres become very short, the cells either die or become senescent, which means that they remain alive but can cause genetic damage. The study's authors noted that their findings "suggest that work-related exhaustion is related to the acceleration of the rate of biological aging." In other words, high levels of stress on the job could be aging you quickly!

But it's not just stress on the job that can whittle away at your telomeres and speed up the aging process. In a groundbreaking study conducted by E. S. Epel, investigators examined the impact of chronic stress on thirty-nine women (ages twenty to fifty) who had been taking care of a chronically ill child for one to twelve years. Nineteen women who had healthy children served as the control group.

When the researchers looked at the telomeres of the women who had chronically ill children, their telomeres were shorter than those of the control women. In fact, the longer the women with ill children had been caregiving, the shorter their telomeres. The researchers also found that the women's perception of stress also affected telomere length. Women who perceived themselves to be under a great deal of stress had telomeres that were similar to someone a full decade older when compared with women who perceived themselves to have the lowest level of stress.

This finding regarding the perception of stress is important to keep in mind when you read step 3 on how to relax and free your mind!

STRESS AND AGING

I have already mentioned that stress can whittle away at your telomeres, which speeds up the aging process and shortens the life span. But stress has other ways of making you age faster. For example:

- A 2011 study of people age sixty-five and older found that stress associated with financial worries was causing a growing number of adults in this age group to turn to drinking alcohol or smoking, or to increase how much they engaged in these habits.

- Stress takes a big toll on your skin. The appearance of fine lines and wrinkles can be a direct consequence of chronic stress—your face reveals all! Elevated cortisol levels dehydrate the body, which leads to premature wrinkling. In *The Wrinkle Cure* by Dr. Nicholas Perricone, he notes that elevated cortisol levels not only age the skin through dehydration, but also because they foster a decline in the production of collagen and elastin, substances necessary for skin health.

- While mild to moderate stress experienced during learning can have an invigorating effect on memory, excessive or chronic stress can be seriously detrimental to the memory process.

- Chronic stress plays a major part in diseases often associated with aging, including heart disease, stroke, and cancer.

- Stress depletes nutrients that have an important role in fighting stress, which include B vitamins and magnesium. Not only does the depletion of these nutrients make it harder to fight stress, but a deficiency can contribute to cognitive problems (e.g., ability to concentrate) and graying of your hair.

- Stress is a major contributor to sleep problems, including insomnia. Perhaps you could get away with not sleeping well when you were young, but as you get older, insufficient sleep can make you look older very quickly, as well as have a detrimental effect on your cognitive functioning.

The bottom line: stress can add lines to your face and silver to your hair while subtracting years from your life.

STRESS AND PREGNANCY

If you are pregnant or have been pregnant, you know that pregnancy is a stressful time of life. Although you may be thrilled with the prospect of having a child, pregnancy places physical and emotional demands (stressors) on women; for example, hormone fluctuations cause mood changes while morning sickness, weight gain, headaches, back pain, swelling, and other physical changes can cause significant discomfort and the need to make lifestyle changes—all of which are stressful. In addition, women may have worries about the health of the fetus, financial concerns, trepidation about labor and delivery, and other issues surrounding pregnancy, all of which add to the stress burden.

Women who experience chronic stress during pregnancy are at risk for additional health problems both before and after delivery. Stress-related health problems, such as high blood pressure and heart disease, present during pregnancy, can increase a woman's chances of premature birth or a low-birthweight infant. Stress also compromises the immune system and increases the chances of postpartum depression.

In a study presented in October 2012 in New Orleans at the annual meeting of the Society for Neuroscience, researchers reported that rats who experienced chronic stress during pregnancy did not have an increase in brain cell structures that improve behavioral flexibility and cognitive function while unstressed rat mothers enjoyed this benefit. The bottom line was that the stressed rats displayed behaviors seen in human mothers who have postpartum depression, while the unstressed rats did not. According to the study's lead author, Benedetta Leuner of Ohio State University, the stressed rats "don't have the capacity for brain plasticity that the unstressed mothers do, and somehow that's contributing to their susceptibility to depression."

Although pregnancy is a temporary condition, stress during this critical time of a woman's life should be addressed as quickly and safely as possible. If you are pregnant and are experiencing significant levels of stress, you should talk to a health-care professional as soon as possible and discuss natural, safe steps you can take to reduce your exposure to stress, including many of the options discussed in part 2 of this book.

STRESS AND FOOD

Cynthia stands at the kitchen counter, chewing her food with gusto. No, not because she is conscientious about making sure she thoroughly masticates every morsel, and not because she is hungry. It's nearly midnight and Cynthia can't sleep—again—and as she has done on far too many nights, she gets out of bed, starts to pace, and ends up in front of the refrigerator or kitchen cabinets, reaching not for a cup of comforting chamomile tea but for crackers or cookies or leftover pizza.

Although Cynthia may think she's finding comfort in her midnight raids for high-carbohydrate foods, instead she is fueling her chronic stress, and the kindling is considerable. Her six-year-old son, Jason, has autism, and she has been struggling with school officials for months about his behavior in the classroom. Melanie, her ten-year-old daughter, is doing well in school, but recently has been relentlessly begging for expensive clothes that Cynthia simply can't afford on her salary. And with personnel cutbacks at the office, where Cynthia is a production manager, she has had to work longer hours, even bring work home on the weekends. She's exhausted and has been fighting a cold for months and has recurring headaches.

Cynthia's chronic state of anxiety keeps her stress hormones (corticotropin-releasing hormone and glucocorticoids) elevated. Glucocorticoids are junk food junkies, and they prompt the desire for the so-called comfort foods: those fatty, salty, sweet items you crave. Why do you want these foods so much? Because glucocorticoids trigger a system in the brain called the ventral tegmental area, which is also stimulated by cocaine and other abused drugs. Although the lure of potato chips and chocolate chip cookies may not be as strong as the addictive power of heroin, the basic process is the same.

Wait, there's more. When you seek stress relief in sweet, high-fat foods such as chocolate ice cream or cherry pie, the body releases more natural painkillers called endorphins, which in turn rev up the release of dopamine. This is the same pattern followed by drugs of abuse. Research conducted by Elissa Epel from the University of California, San Francisco (and one of the pioneers in telomere research as well), and others has shown that the release of glucocorticoids triggered by eating comfort foods prompts a big release of dopamine, which in turn stimulates you to want more comfort food.

This vicious cycle keeps chronic stress alive, but it also works at not keeping you well or healthy. The intake of unhealthy foods and extra calories pack on the pounds and fat, especially around the belly, which stimulates even more glucocorticoids to be released. In addition, the combination of stress, bad food, excess glucocorticoids, and fat plays havoc with your blood sugar levels, increase your risk of heart disease and diabetes, and sets your moods swinging.

According to Nora D. Volkow, MD, director of the National Institute on Drug Abuse, the addictive quality of drugs is believed to be related to their ability to "increase the concentration of dopamine in the brain," and when that hormone keeps being released, "the number of receptors starts to decrease." When dopamine receptors decline and then give out, the ability to experience pleasure goes as well and depression takes over.

STRESS, INSULIN, AND DIABETES

Type 2 diabetes is an epidemic in the United States and many other places around the world. As of 2012, the World Health Organization estimated that 220 million people around the world had the disease. Unfortunately, type 2 diabetes is not a benign condition. Having the disease is associated with a two- to fourfold increased risk you will experience a coronary heart problem, an increased risk for diabetes complications (e.g., eye disease [retinopathy], kidney problems [nephropathy], nerve problems [neuropathy]), and a doubled risk for depression.

One positive aspect of type 2 diabetes, however, is that it is a lifestyle disease, which means it is basically caused by—and therefore can be prevented and successfully managed and even reversed—factors that can be modified, such as diet, exercise, and weight. Stress is also one of those factors.

According to a report from the European Depression in Diabetes (EDID) Research Consortium in 2010, even though the exact causes of type 2 diabetes are not known, it seems clear that depression is a risk factor, and it's also been established that chronic emotional stress is a risk factor for the development of depression. The authors of the consortium also noted that based on research results, depression, emotional stress and anxiety, sleeping difficulties, hostility, and anger are associated with an increased risk for developing type 2 diabetes.

In addition, chronic stress can cause your body to develop insulin resistance, which means your cells are unable to respond properly to the overproduction of insulin due to elevated blood sugar levels caused by stress. The result is that your appetite can increase while your body's ability to burn fat declines, and you gain weight.

So what does this mean to you? First of all, no one wants to develop diabetes, so if you have other risk factors for the disease (e.g., overweight/obesity, insulin resistance, high triglycerides, family history of diabetes, among others), the presence of chronic stress in your life is not helping. Even if you don't seem to be at risk for type 2 diabetes, living with chronic stress still is not a healthy situation. The bottom line is, it's in your best interest to reduce or eliminate the stress in your life.

WOMEN, STRESS, AND DIABETES

- A Swedish study looked at the impact of work stress and low emotional support on the prospect of developing type 2 diabetes among middle-aged men and women. More than 33,000 adults were included in the study, and none of them had type 2 diabetes when they entered the study. After an average of 5.4 years, 191 individuals were diagnosed with the disease. The investigators found that stressful work circumstances and low emotional support were associated with future type 2 diabetes among women, but not among men. Even after the authors made allowances for risk factors associated with type 2 diabetes, such as body mass index, the risk for the women remained the same.

- What about young females? Does stress have an effect on whether they might develop type 2 diabetes? A 2012 report from Athens University Medical School suggests the answer is yes. The authors reported specifically on the impact of stress during childhood and adolescence and reported that chronic stress "may lead to the development of or may exacerbate . . . anxiety disorders, depression, obesity, and the metabolic syndrome," which is the predecessor of type 2 diabetes, they also pointed out that "chronic alterations in cortisol [a stress hormone] secretion in children may affect . . . early onset obesity, metabolic syndrome, and type 2 diabetes mellitus."

PART 2

Manage (and Banish) Your Stress in 7 Easy Steps

Now that you have identified your stressors and realize there are ways to eliminate them (utilizing the DROP—Delegate, Reduce, Organize, and/or Prioritize—approach), and know what stressors can do to your body and mind, it's time to make a plan. To effectively manage and banish your stress, you need to make a personal commitment to achieve that goal. To help you with that process, the chapters throughout this section will help you learn about dozens of ways to handle and bust through stress and nurture yourself, including hands-on techniques, nutrition and natural remedies, personal and creative development, relaxation skills, movement therapies, social outreach, and professional assistance. At the same time, you should remain ever mindful to find ways to incorporate DROP elements into your stress-management plan.

It's essential to have a wide spectrum of stress-reducing options at your disposal so you can launch a multifaceted attack. That's because the stress in your life has many sources and triggers, and so you need to face them with a variety of softening tools. It's also reassuring to know that there are other things you can do when something may not work out! You want to have many options from which to choose so that your selection process doesn't create additional stress.

As you read through the following chapters, you will develop your stress reduction plan. First, check out the introductory box at the start of each chapter, which lets you know what is covered in that chapter. Do you see ideas that pique your interest? Great! Read about them, and if you are still intrigued, add it (or them) to your list. Continue on through all the chapters in the same way. Hint: you don't have to check out or read the chapters in order. Scan the chapter titles and start with the one that most captures your attention.

Every woman's journey through step 2 will be different: you may find some interesting options right away, try them, and begin to construct a stress-reducing plan that works for you very quickly. Or you may go through several or all of the chapters, pick and choose approaches to try and either add to your plan or discard options that don't work for you. The choice is yours. It is recommended, however, that you remain open-minded and select several stress-reducing strategies to include in your plan so you can attack your stress from all sides.

Once you have a plan, write it down and post it somewhere conspicuous: on your refrigerator, bathroom mirror, inside the front door, on your dashboard. Remind yourself of your commitment to reduce stress in your life! Let your family know you are on a mission and that your mission is good for everyone concerned. If you want, let them be involved in your stress reduction journey. In fact, including your spouse/partner, children, and friends in your plan is the Delegate part of DROP, which you read about in chapter 2. But the ultimate journey will be your own.

STEP 1

Hands-On Stress Busters

Touch has the power to heal, and that includes its ability to put the brakes on stress and how it can run away with your life. This chapter discusses various types of hands-on stress busters, some of which you can do yourself, some you can ask a partner or friend to do for you, or some that may be done by a professional, including acupressure, acupuncture, massage, Reiki, and Zero Balancing. When applicable, there are instructions on how women can do the therapy themselves or with a friend, plus details about how each of the approaches works to reduce stress. Remember DROP and make one of these stress reducers a Priority and Delegate some task so you can make time for yourself because you deserve it!

ACUPRESSURE

Imagine you are sitting in another one of those long, boring staff meetings, knowing there is a pile of work on your desk that you should be doing. You're beginning to feel the tension increasing in your neck, between your shoulder blades, and between your eyes. You want to relax, release the stress and tension, but you can't close your eyes and meditate, can't start practicing deep breathing, so what can you do?

Or perhaps your kids are bickering—again and still!—in the other room, and you're trying to prepare dinner after a long day at the office. You'd love to take a long walk to let go of your stress, but you can't get away. You need a shot of stress relief.

Acupressure is an option. The ancient Chinese healing art of acupressure is something you can do yourself without the need for any materials—just your own fingertips. Acupressure can relieve tension, enhance circulation, and reduce pain and stress when pressure is applied to selected acupressure points, which you can learn to do yourself. As an added bonus, you can do acupressure just about anywhere—while sitting or standing, driving, waiting in line, lying in bed, or making breakfast.

Acupressure is similar to acupuncture in that it is based on the concept of the body's vital life energy, or chi (qi). While acupuncture uses needles to tap into the vital life energy at designated points (called acupoints or trigger points) on the body, acupressure uses finger pressure, and the same points can be treated. Tension tends to congregate around acupoints, and so when you apply pressure to these points, muscles that have tightened because of stress, fatigue, or tension can relax and thus allow blood to reach them and deliver healing oxygen and nutrients. At the same time, any toxins that have accumulated in the muscles can be released and eliminated from the body.

Acupressure can be helpful on its own, but you can enhance its benefits if you combine it with other simple stress reduction techniques (also discussed in this book), such as deep breathing, stretching, guided imagery, and meditation. If you add acupressure to your stress-management plan, consider pairing it with other complementary techniques for maximum results.

Six Acupressure Points

You can apply pressure to any of the following acupoints to help you relax and calm your mind. In each case, apply pressure for one minute and use a very small, circular massaging motion with your thumb tip on the point. You should apply enough pressure to feel a comfortable level of pain. Repeat on the opposite side of the body, when applicable. Feel free to use acupressure throughout the day whenever you feel stressed.

- **Point 1.** Clench your left hand so the tendons in your forearm stick out. Starting at the crease that goes across your wrist at the base of your left hand, use the thumb on your right hand to measure two thumb widths toward your elbow. The acupoint is located between the two tendons. Relax your hand, then use the tip of your right thumb to press the point and massage it. Pressure on this point may also relieve insomnia and an upset stomach.

- **Point 2.** This point can be found on the crease on your wrist, as mentioned in point 1. Place your thumb from your opposite hand on the crease directly in line with your little finger, just inside the edge of your wrist bone. Pressure on this point may also help relieve insomnia and heart palpitations.

- **Point 3.** To find this point, place your left hand palm down. Place the thumb of your right hand on the third finger of your left hand, immediately above the cuticle and to the right of the nail.

- **Point 4.** This acupoint is located in the flat area of your outer ear called the fossa, which is the widest part of your outer ear. Place your index finger inside your ear on the point and your thumb on the back of your fossa directly behind your finger. This allows you to massage both sides of the point. Pressure on this point is reportedly one of the most effective in relieving stress and feelings of being overwhelmed.

- **Point 5.** In a small hollow area below the head of your collarbone, immediately adjacent to your breastbone, there is a great stress-reducing acupoint. Traditional Chinese healers call this point Elegant Mansion, and it is effective for relieving stress, opening up your breathing passages (helpful in stressful situations), and can also clear chest congestion. Be sure to treat this point on both sides of your breastbone.

- **Point 6.** This instruction is actually for two acupoints to be pressed simultaneously. One is between your eyebrows, immediately above the bridge of your nose. Use your right middle fingertip to press this point while using the middle-finger tip of your left hand to press and massage the point in the center of your breastbone, between your nipples and directly in line with them. If you are experiencing a great deal of stress, the acupoint on your chest may feel sore.

Acupressure Studies

- Being transported to a hospital in an ambulance is a stressful situation, and it was the setting for a randomized, blind study that evaluated the use of acupressure applied to the relaxation point in the ear (seventeen patients) versus pressure applied to a sham point (nineteen patients). The patients who received the true acupressure reported significantly less stress and anxiety than did patients in the sham group on arrival to the hospital, concerning pain during treatment, and regarding treatment outcomes.

- Health-care workers and hospital staff (doctors, nurses, clinicians, administrators) face lots of stress on the job, and so a study was done in which employees of a military hospital were offered a chance to visit an on-site wellness clinic one day per week. They could choose one or more stress-reducing therapies: ear acupuncture, acupressure, and/or Zero Balancing, which involves massage of acupressure points along with stretching (see "Zero Balancing"). Based on the responses from participants after their first and repeat visits (total, 2,756 surveys), 97.9 percent agreed or strongly agreed they felt more relaxed, 94.5 percent said they felt less stress, and 84.3 percent said they had more energy as a result of their visits. Among those who had five or more visits, 59 percent to 85 percent strongly agreed they had better relations with their coworkers, more compassion for patients, improved mood, and better sleep.

ACUPUNCTURE

The ancient Chinese art of acupuncture has become integrated into conventional medicine more than ever before, and for good reason: scientific studies show that it is effective for a number of common problems, including pain, fatigue, insomnia, and stress. Since it's not uncommon for stress to be accompanied by at least one of the first three mentioned factors, it's good to know acupuncture may take care of all these challenges.

According to ancient Chinese philosophy, the body harbors two opposing forces called yin and yang. When your yin and yang are balanced, you are healthy. To stay in balance, the life force or energy force called chi or qi that travels throughout the body along channels called meridians needs to flow freely. If something blocks the flow of energy, the result can be illness, be it physical, emotional, spiritual, or all three.

Placement of extremely thin needles into various acupoints along the meridians can free up blocked chi and restore energy flow. Professional acupuncture practitioners know exactly which points (there are about two thousand!) to address to promote the body's natural healing abilities and to return balance.

More and more Western health-care providers are embracing acupuncture as a complementary treatment, even though the explanation for why it can be effective differs from the Chinese perspective. Western practitioners are apt to say acupuncture works because it stimulates the central nervous system and triggers the release of substances (e.g., endorphins, neurotransmitters) that have a role in regulating bodily functions, reducing pain, and enhancing the immune system. (See "Acupuncture Studies" for some examples of scientific studies of acupuncture.)

Acupuncture requires a qualified professional, so this is one stress-management technique you shouldn't do on your own. Even occasional acupuncture sessions, especially if you also practice other complementary stress-reduction techniques, can provide significant relief. If there is an acupuncture school in your area, it may offer sessions at a reduced rate or on a sliding scale.

ACUPUNCTURE STUDIES

* An August 2012 study published in *Complementary Therapies in Clinical Practice* explored how forty-seven patients who visited their general practitioner responded to six acupuncture treatments of forty-five minutes each. All the participants completed a questionnaire called the Measure Your Medical Outcome Profile both before the first acupuncture treatment and after the last. Overall they reported a significant improvement in various areas, including a reduc-

continued

tion in stress and pain, reduced use of medication, and an improved quality of life.

- Twenty-five medical students were the subjects in a study that evaluated the use of acupuncture on stress-related symptoms, such as depression, anxiety, burnout, and sleep disorders. Twelve students received twenty minutes of electroacupuncture once a week for eight weeks while thirteen students received no treatment. All the students completed questionnaires that related to each of the stress-related symptoms. Students who received acupuncture showed significant improvements in depression, burnout, physical health, and emotional exhaustion when compared with controls. Sleep also improved: 75 percent of students in the acupuncture group had good sleep quality compared with 23.1 percent of control students.

- Acupuncture appeared to have a positive impact on stress in women who underwent embryo transfer. At the University of Pittsburgh, fifty-seven infertile women scheduled to undergo embryo transfer were assigned to have the procedure either with or without acupuncture as part of their standard care. The researchers found that women who received acupuncture had lower stress scores than did women who did not have acupuncture; and women in the acupuncture group had a pregnancy rate of 64.7 percent compared with 42.5 percent among women who did not receive acupuncture.

MASSAGE

Massage: just hearing the word may prompt you to release the tension lurking in your neck and shoulders. Yet what exactly comes to mind when you think of massage? Depending on your experience with massage, whether it's personal or just what you've seen in movies or heard about from others, it can include about eighty different therapy styles. These various techniques are distinguished by a variety of methods and pressures applied by a therapist using her fingers, hands, elbows, and perhaps even her feet and forearms.

Massage has become accepted as a significantly effective way to experience relief from stress and anxiety, heal injuries, enhance circulation, and promote overall health. From the locker room to the boardroom, or a massage table in an exclusive spa to a massage chair at a health fair, massage is a sought-after therapy. According to the American Massage Therapy Association, 18 percent of adults (about 38 million) in the United States had a massage at least once between July 2010 and July 2011. The main reasons for seeking a massage are medical problems and stress.

Although there are dozens of types of massage, certain styles are better suited for reducing stress and tension. The most common type of massage is Swedish massage, which involves four basic strokes:

- Effleurage: long, smooth strokes that relax soft tissue

- Friction: deeper, circular strokes that help enhance blood flow and break up any scar tissue

- Petrissage: kneading or squeezing strokes that are typically used after effleurage

- Tapotement: short, alternating taps performed with the fingers, edge of the hands, or cupped hands

Overall, Swedish massage relaxes and energizes the top layers of muscles, leaving the recipient feeling "limp and lively at the same time," as one woman likes to describe it. Practitioners of Swedish massage also include gentle movement of the joints, which promotes flexibility.

Another common type of massage is reflexology, a technique that involves using the fingertips and thumbs to stimulate specific areas of the feet. (Naturally, a simple whole foot massage feels great as well!) In reflexology, these areas are believed to correspond to specific parts of the body. When these spots are massaged, therefore, they can stimulate and promote well-being, including relief from tension and stress.

Getting a Massage

If you are able to enjoy the services of a professional massage therapist, even if it's only occasionally, then I encourage you to do so. Massage therapy schools typically offer massages given by their students, at a reduced rate. Many communities also have classes taught by massage professionals, where you or you and a partner can learn how to give each other a massage.

One of the beauties of massage is that you can quickly learn to give yourself a massage or have a partner do it for you. Here are a few examples of self-massage that you can do at home, at work, or even a few you can do while waiting in line. You may want to enhance your massage experience by using essential oils, which are discussed in step 4.

Self-massage for tension and headache

- Place your thumbs on your cheekbones near your ears. Use your fingertips to gently press and rub your temples at the soft spot between your ear and the corner of your eye.

- Use firm pressure while also slowly making circular motions, gradually moving your fingers up along your hairline. When your fingers meet in the center of your forehead, continue to massage your scalp and forehead. Also take slow, deep breaths as you do the massage, gently releasing each breath.

Self-massage for neck tension

If you sit at a desk or in front of a computer for hours, this self-massage technique can work wonders for relieving stress and tension in your neck.

- While in a seated position, place your hands over the tops of your shoulders. Slowly exhale as you allow your head to fall back and squeeze your fingers toward your palms, moving up the muscles of your back and shoulders toward your neck.

- Rest your elbows on your desk and let your head drop forward in a comfortable position. Use your fingertips to massage your neck along your shoulders to the base of your skull. Make firm, circular motions, massaging the muscles that lie on either side of your spine.

- Now place both palms on the back of your head and intertwine your fingers. Allow your head to fall forward to a comfortable position, while also letting the weight of your elbows pull your head down. Feel the muscles of your neck and upper back gently stretch and release their tension.

Self-massage for tense shoulder muscles

You need a tennis ball or solid rubber ball to help you with this self-massage technique.

- Stand about eighteen inches from a wall and place your feet hip distance apart.

- Drop slowly into a partial squat position with your buttocks against the wall.

- Lean forward and place the ball at the top of your left shoulder.

- Stand up slowly, inching your way until you are standing fully upright. Press your back and shoulders against the wall and allow the ball to slowly roll down the muscles along the side of your spine. If you reach an uncomfortable spot, stop and wait for the pain to subside.

- Reverse your movement by slowing squatting down and allowing the ball to roll back up to the top of your shoulder muscles.

- Switch sides: place the ball at the top of your right shoulder and repeat the self-massage.

STUDIES OF MASSAGE AND STRESS REDUCTION

- Nurses experience a great deal of on-the-job stress (and probably off the job as well!), and so they were the subjects in this Mayo Clinic study. Thirty-eight nurses were offered weekly fifteen-minute chair massages for ten weeks. After ten weeks, scores on both of the stress tests had declined and self-assessment and symptom scores had improved. The authors concluded that massage reduced stress-related symptoms in the nurses.

- What effect does massage have on stress responses in healthy individuals? This study decided to find out in twenty-two volunteers (eleven men, eleven women) with an average age of 28.2 years. All the participants underwent massage in a crossover study, which means all the participants were tested after experiencing eighty minutes of massage and also after a controlled state (resting without massage). After only five minutes of massage, the participants experienced a significant reduction in heart rate, which indicated a reduced stress response. As the massage continued, other stress-reduction factors were noted, such as heart rate variability, insulin levels, and cortisol levels.

- People who are waiting to undergo an invasive cardiovascular procedure can be expected to feel stressed, and so a study was conducted to

continued

see if massage therapy could reduce stress, anxiety, and pain in patients scheduled for such events. A total of 130 patients were offered either twenty minutes of massage therapy at least thirty minutes before their cardiovascular procedure or standard preprocedure care. The results indicate that massage is an effective way to reduce stress, pain, and anxiety before cardiovascular procedures.

Does Massage Lower Cortisol Levels?

One way scientists can determine if a technique or medication is reducing stress is to look at its impact on cortisol levels. Thus far, research on the effect of massage on cortisol levels has produced conflicting results. For example, a 2010 study reported from Germany explored how massage affected stress perception and mood among thirty-four women with breast cancer. The women were randomly assigned to receive either biweekly thirty-minute massage sessions (seventeen women) along with their routine health care, or routine health care without massage (seventeen women).

The women completed stress and mood questionnaires and had blood samples taken to determine cortisol levels before, at the end of the trial, and six weeks after the trial. Compared with women in the control group, those who had received massage reported significantly fewer mood problems (especially anger, anxious depression, and tiredness). In addition, cortisol levels were significantly reduced after massage therapy compared with before therapy.

In a subsequent study conducted at the University of Wisconsin, an investigative team reviewed the literature on whether massage can lower cortisol levels. Overall the reviewers concluded that massage therapy has a "very small" impact on cortisol and that it's likely that the reason for the "well-established and statistically larger beneficial effects" of massage therapy are associated with other mechanisms besides cortisol.

REIKI

Reiki is a stress-reduction technique that promotes relaxation and healing using the "laying on of hands." The "secret" of Reiki can be found in its name. It is composed of two Japanese words: "rei" means "God's wisdom or the higher power," while "ki" means "life force energy." This is the same life force (chi or qi, as discussed in the section on acupressure and acupuncture) that flows through the body along meridians or channels. This life force also flows around the body in an energy field called the aura.

When this life force is blocked, a person's health (physical, emotional, mental, and/or spiritual) suffers. Therefore, when you receive Reiki from a practitioner, you receive spiritually guided energy that promotes and recharges the flow of your life force energy. Reiki can be used safely and easily with any other type of medical or alternative therapies.

How to Experience Reiki

Reiki is spiritual in nature, but it is not a religion, and people do not need to be spiritual to receive Reiki or to benefit from it. However, it's important for people who practice and give Reiki to behave in ways that promote balance and harmony. If you want to try Reiki, practitioners often can be found through holistic health food stores, spiritual resource centers, and on the Internet.

Although receiving Reiki from a professional or someone else who has learned Reiki can be a great experience, some people learn to do Reiki for themselves. Typically it takes about eight to twelve hours of in-person training to learn Reiki, and then you can be ready to help yourself (and others if you choose) to relieve stress and restore balance to your life.

Lisa, a fifty-three-year-old software analyst, turned to Reiki several years ago when she was looking for a way to help manage the stress from her job, which was affecting every other part of her life. "I was recently divorced, and the demands of my job were making it difficult to get my life back together. I desperately needed to keep my job to support myself, and the stress of worrying just made it even harder to cope."

A friend took Lisa to a lecture about Reiki at a local health fair, and after hearing the Reiki master talk about the benefits of the healing practice and especially how Lisa could learn to give herself Reiki, she decided to sign up for the ten hours of training. After learning Reiki and using it on herself, she decided she wanted to learn more, and eventually she went on to the second stage of training and plans to become a Reiki master.

"When I learned Reiki, it opened up whole new possibilities for me," says Lisa. "I now feel like I have some control of my life and my way in the world. When demands from work and from my kids build up, Reiki is always there to help me center myself, restore my balance. And because Reiki has helped me so much, I decided to learn more and help others, and that is so rewarding."

Research studies have been conducted on the benefits of Reiki for stress, anxiety, pain, and other health issues. For example:

- A 2011 study published in *Critical Care Nursing* reported that Reiki can "relieve pain and anxiety and reduce symptoms of stress such as elevated blood pressure and pulse rates."

- Work-related stress is a major reason why registered nurses burn out and quit. A study conducted at Boston Medical Center evaluated the impact of Reiki on seventeen registered nurses who were taught Reiki. The investigators found that the practice of self-administered Reiki more often led to reduced perceived stress levels.

ZERO BALANCING

In the 1970s, Fritz Smith, MD, who was a pioneer in integrative medicine, developed a mind-body therapy called Zero Balancing, which combines finger pressure and gentle traction to restore balance in the body. Picture in your mind a bathroom scale, the type that has a dial with numbers and an arm that points to the weight. After you step on and off the scale often over time, the scale tends to become slightly off balance: it no longer returns and resets to zero when you step off the scale. You need to return the scale to zero.

Similarly, life is full of situations and events that can cause stress, interfere with your natural state of health, and throw you off balance. Zero Balancing can help restore the right harmony of energy and structure in the body, bringing you back to a state of relaxation. It is not a self-therapy, and so you would need to find a Zero Balancing practitioner to facilitate the balancing process.

How Zero Balancing Works

The basic concept of Zero Balancing is that both the physical body and the energy body can be treated together using "educated touch," which is also referred to as "interface." Practitioners of Zero Balancing have been trained to have both a tactile (touch) and intellectual understanding of a person's energy. During a Zero Balancing session, which lasts about thirty to forty-five minutes, practitioners follow a general treatment approach to work with the energy and structures of the body. Both finger pressure and traction are applied to various areas of soft tissue and to key joints and bones to reintroduce balance and relaxation. A basic foundation of Zero Balancing is the concept that bones, ligaments, and other connective tissues conduct energy, and that the combination of finger pressure and traction releases energy flow throughout the musculoskeletal system.

This release of energy clears any blockages in the flow of vital energy and helps to relieve stress and muscle tension, improve posture, enhance vitality and flexibility, and promote overall well-being. Zero Balancing also works at the emotional, mental, and spiritual levels, releasing memories and stress patterns stored in the body's tissues that hamper a person's ability to thrive and grow.

Studies of Zero Balancing

The wellness clinic at a U.S. Department of Defense hospital was the setting for a study of the effectiveness of a weekly on-site complementary medicine program that included Zero Balancing, ear acupuncture, and acupressure. Individuals invited to participate included nurses, doctors, hospital support staff, and administrators, and they could choose any one or more of the offerings.

All the participants were asked to complete surveys after their first visit and repeat visits. From a total of 2,756 surveys, the study's authors found that most participants agreed or strongly agreed that they were more relaxed (97.9 percent), felt less stress (94.5 percent), had more energy (84.3 percent), and experienced less pain (78.8 percent) because of attending the sessions. Participants also reported that the benefits were sustained and improved by repeat visits for therapy, and that they had a positive impact on stress at work.

In the journal *Holistic Nursing Practice,* Sallie Stoltz Denner explains that even though Zero Balancing is "not yet considered an evidence-based technique," practitioners have used it successfully for stress conditions, and that dramatic results have been obtained when it's been used along with hypnosis for depression and post-traumatic stress syndrome.

Finding a Zero Balancing Practitioner

Some acupuncture therapists, chiropractors, massage therapists, nurses, occupational therapists, osteopaths, physical therapists, craniosacral therapists, and psychotherapists, among other professionals, have been trained in Zero Balancing. When looking for a qualified practitioner, ask if he or she has been certified. Individuals who have received certification have participated in at least 175 hours of continuing education, one-on-one mentoring, and performance evaluations.

STEP 2

Move Away from Stress

Human beings have been designed to move. We even move when we sleep (have you been kicked or elbowed by your bed partner lately?). Physical activity supports and nurtures every part of the body, from increasing blood flow to strengthening and toning muscles, stretching ligaments and tendons, and promoting strong bones. You need to keep moving to energize the life force.

But physical activity also is important for other reasons: movement completes the circle of life and is tied in to your emotional, mental, and spiritual essence as well as your physical being. One of the exciting things about movement is variety: whether you walk, run, row, do aerobics, swim, stretch, do yoga or tai chi, all of them are positive, life supporting, and stress reducing, and they have an impact at a cellular level. Movement also has a positive effect on stress and anxiety.

In a survey called Stress in America, conducted by the American Psychological Association and published in *Psychology Today,* 1,226 adults were questioned about their stress levels. On a scale of 1 (little or no stress) to 10 (high stress), the researchers found that the average stress levels had declined from 6.2 in 2007 to 5.2 in 2011. The age group showing the most decline was among baby boomers, with a drop from 4.5 in 2007 to 3.4 in 2011. According to Teri L. Bourdeau, professor at the Oklahoma State University Center for Health Sciences, the findings of the survey "may have to do with the increased engagement in physically challenging and engaging activities."

Does physical activity help banish stress? That's the question I asked fifty-seven-year-old Carmella, as she was making her way down the boardwalk in Wildwood, New Jersey. "When I'm power walking, I feel like I'm shedding my anxiety and stress as I walk, leaving it all behind me. That's how I envision it," she said. "I'm out here nearly every day, rain or shine, because it's my tension fighter, my fix. Sorry I can't stop to talk, I just need to walk!" Carmella said as she moved swiftly through the early morning strollers.

To reduce, manage, and banish stress, it's important to keep moving, and to do it daily. So organize your schedule and get ready to make movement a Priority in your life. This chapter offers some suggestions to make it possible.

AEROBIC EXERCISE

Did you know that whenever you walk, jog, row, ride a bike, jump rope, or engage in other forms of aerobic exercise, you are doing your body, mind, and spirit lots of great favors? For example, aerobic exercise is an effective way to burn calories, lose weight, and/or maintain a healthy weight. Your heart and circulatory system become stronger and more efficient, and even your skin will be healthier because of improved blood flow. Lung capacity can improve, and more oxygen reaches the brain, which can improve your ability to concentrate and release stress. When you keep moving, your muscles also can get stronger and more toned.

And there's more. Aerobic exercise can help banish stress and anxiety, and much of that benefit comes from the release of endorphins that occurs with exercise. Endorphins are natural biochemicals that act as neurotransmitters and help people feel more positive and calm, and they also help reduce pain. Although you don't need to do vigorous exercise to enjoy the advantages of endorphins, more intense activity helps increase the rate at which endorphins are sent into your circulatory system. In addition, exercise helps reduce levels of the stress hormones cortisol and adrenaline.

A quick note on dance is necessary here. Although dancing is a wonderful aerobic exercise, I did not include it in this chapter because dance also is a great means of creative expression. Therefore, dance is discussed in step 5, "Express Yourself."

Aerobics and Telomeres

You might remember our discussion of telomeres, the "caps" that protect the ends of your chromosomes from damage that can be caused by chronic stress. Scientists have shown that aerobic exercise can help protect the telomeres.

In fact, researchers did a study that involved stressed but otherwise healthy postmenopausal women and compared telomere length among women who exercised vigorously with those who were sedentary. They found that the women who did not exercise had a fifteenfold increased risk of having short telomeres, leading them to conclude that "vigorous physical activity appears to protect those experiencing high stress by buffering its relationship with TL [telomere length]."

Get Moving!

It's recommended you engage in aerobic exercise at least four days a week, and preferably more. If you make it a Priority and ink it into your daily calendar, then you are much more likely to do it, and you will be so glad you did! Aerobic exercise allows you time for yourself or, if you prefer, you can share your walk, jog, aerobics, or tennis with a friend. If you team up with a buddy, then you can support each other not only with exercise, but also companionship, which is another stress reducer.

Here are a few suggestions for how to incorporate stress-reducing aerobic exercise into your life:

- Have a dog? Walk it! Don't have a dog? Ask your neighbor or a family member if you can take their dog for a walk or jog.

- Park several blocks away from where you work and walk (only if it's safe, of course).

- Use part or all of your lunch break to walk.

- March in place while watching television. You can also add hand weights to increase your exercise effort.

- Do aerobic exercises at home using exercise tapes or CDs. If you have small children, get them involved as well and show them exercise can be fun.

- Drag out that bicycle from the back of the garage and bike around the neighborhood (again, if it is safe).

- Take dance lessons. Zumba, salsa, ballroom, jazz, tap; there are lots of possibilities. Check out low-cost and even free lessons at senior centers, community centers, fitness centers, and schools. I discuss the benefits of dance in step 5 on releasing your creative spirit.

- Do mall walking. Some women live in areas that are not safe or otherwise appropriate for walking, or the weather may be too harsh. Some malls have walking programs that allow groups or individuals to walk inside malls before the stores are open.

- Start a neighborhood or workplace walking program. Hey, you're not the only one who needs to work off some stress!

"I have a calendar, and I write down my three aerobic classes every week," says Becky. "The funny thing is, I really enjoy these classes, and they make me feel great. But if I don't write them down and make them a priority, then I tend to let them go because I get so wrapped up with my work or doing errands for my kids. When I do this for myself, I feel better about my work, myself, and my family. I figure that's a pretty good deal!"

ALEXANDER TECHNIQUE

According to *The Complete Guide to the Alexander Technique*, which is touted as "the most comprehensive source for information about the Alexander Technique worldwide," this movement approach is "a way of learning how you can get rid of harmful tension in your body." Part of the concept of the Alexander Technique is that it shows you how to change your movements in your everyday activities so you can achieve balance and release unnecessary stress and tension.

The Alexander Technique is not an exercise: it is a re-education of how to move with more freedom, coordination, support, and ease. The end result is less stress on your body and mind, more energy, better posture, and an overall sense of well-being and calm. You can apply what you learn from Alexander Technique lessons while sitting, standing, lying down, lifting, walking, and just doing routine activities.

What to Expect from Alexander Technique Lessons

You don't need any special clothing or equipment to participate in Alexander Technique lessons, but you will likely feel more at ease if you wear comfortable clothing and shoes. The instructor will observe how you move— walk, sit, stand, perform simple activities—and look at your posture. Then he or she will use their hands on your back, shoulders, neck, and so on to gently guide you toward a more stress-free, balanced way of moving or being still. During this process, instructors also are gathering information about your breathing and movement patterns to better help you make adjustments in your behavior.

Lessons typically last thirty to forty-five minutes, and after a few lessons, you and your instructor will have a better idea of how much work you need to do and how well you will be able to achieve it.

Learning the Alexander Technique

The Alexander Technique is best learned from a professional instructor, but the developer of the approach, F. Matthias Alexander, believed that people could learn the necessary techniques if they carefully followed instructions, which are available in written materials, DVDs, and audiotapes (see the appendix), and dedicated themselves to work at it. Some people take several lessons and then continue to apply what they have learned on a daily basis, reinforcing their work with information from books and tapes or returning occasionally for follow-up or refresher lessons. Some instructors work with students online (via Skype).

The American Society for the Alexander Technique certifies instructors of the Alexander Technique. Certified instructors receive three years of training as well as continuing education. If you are interested in learning more about the Alexander Technique and how it can help you manage and reduce stress, look for a certified instructor to help you get started.

What Experts Say about the Alexander Technique and Stress

A number of studies have been done to evaluate the ability of the Alexander Technique to reduce stress and tension and improve performance. Several decades ago (1960s and 1970s), researcher Frank Pierce Jones at Tufts University used electromyography equipment (which measures muscle response) and showed that the Alexander Technique could result in a marked reduction in stress levels. He explained his findings in a book called *Freedom to Change—The Development and Science of the Alexander Technique* (see appendix).

A much more recent study (2010), conducted at the University of Cincinnati Children's Hospital, verified that surgeons who engaged in the Alexander Technique had improved surgical skills in a shorter period of time, experienced improvement in posture, and had better endurance in their shoulders and trunk (critical for surgeons bent over an operating table!). According to Jack Stern, MD, PhD, of the Neurosurgical Group of Westchester, White Plains, New York, the Alexander Technique "teaches people how to best use their bodies in ordinary action to avoid or reduce unnecessary stress and pain. It enables clients to get better faster and stay better longer."

Think about it: do you want to carry your stress with you in your muscles, bones, and tendons in every move you make? Or would you like to learn how to move, sit, and relax in ways that keep your body and mind in balance while releasing stress?

TAI CHI

Tai chi is a mind-body practice that originated in China as a form of martial arts, but which then evolved into a gentle technique, often referred to as "meditation in motion" or mindful movement. A growing number of studies show that tai chi has numerous health benefits, ranging from improving balance and coordination to enhancing flexibility and concentration and reducing stress and tension.

Naturally we are concerned with the latter benefits, but it's hard to separate them from the overall advantages you can get from practicing tai chi. One of the many good things about tai chi is that it can be practiced by people of any age, and you don't need to be in tip-top shape to enjoy it. People in wheelchairs or those who are recovering from surgery can even do some tai chi movements!

Tai chi is especially helpful for older adults who can benefit from the low-impact, slow-motion exercise. Like yoga, tai chi also involves learning how to breathe naturally and deeply, which enhances the stress-reduction experience.

How Tai Chi Works

Tai chi is based on the concepts of qi (chi; the energy or life force that flows through the body) and yin and yang—the opposing elements that are believed to make up the universe and that must be kept in balance for health and harmony. The practice of tai chi is one way to achieve and support this balance because it focuses on promoting the flow of qi.

People who practice tai chi are taught how to move from one pose or movement (which are often named for animals, such as "white crane spreads its wings" or "part the wild horse mane") to another. These names are helpful when learning tai chi, because they help you remember how to move your hands and arms. They also keep you bound with nature and the natural flow of qi.

There are several forms of tai chi, and among the most popular is one called the simplified twenty-four form tai chi, which involves twenty-four movements that are done

one after the other in a flowing motion. This form is good for beginners and is the one often taught as a beginner's course. Once you learn the steps, you can practice them anytime at home, at the office, or, as some people do, at the beach or park!

Learning Tai Chi

Even though tai chi is generally considered to be a safe activity, you should still check with your health-care provider if you have any medical conditions or musculoskeletal problems, or if you are taking medications that can make you dizzy. You will likely be given the go-ahead, but it still is a good idea to check.

The best way to learn tai chi is to take a class, even if you only attend a few sessions, so you can learn the basics. Another option is to use a video or DVD that shows you all the moves. The advantage of attending a class is that an instructor can help you with your moves and your breathing, which is also an important part of tai chi. Classes are also a positive experience because you can experience the energy of the other participants.

Tai chi classes are popular, and they are often offered at senior centers, community centers, fitness centers, and organizations such as the Arthritis Foundation. If, however, you prefer to learn at home, you can use videos, DVDs, and/or books to help you learn the movements.

Pamela, a seventy-four-year-old retired administrator, started taking tai chi classes while she was a caretaker for her husband, Bob, who had Alzheimer's disease. The stress of caring for Bob and the loneliness she felt had started to have a detrimental effect on her health, which she recognized. Although she had no children to help her with nursing care, she finally turned to her church for respite assistance, and someone came and stayed with her husband several hours a week so she could take tai chi classes and run errands.

"The tai chi classes were a lifesaver," she said. "I literally felt like I could fly when I learned how to do the movements. Now I do them at home, even though I still attend classes at least once a week at the senior center in my town. I even do my tai chi at home for my husband, who seems to really enjoy watching me!"

Tai Chi Studies

Tai chi is such a popular form of alternative therapy, and it has been studied extensively, especially for help with balance, arthritis pain, and stress reduction. In the latter category, here are the results of a few studies that illustrate how beneficial tai chi can be.

In a study from Wake Forest University, the authors reported on the experience of nurses (who typically experience a high level of stress) with stress-reduction methods. Of 342 study participants surveyed, 99 percent said they used one or more mind-body approaches to reduce stress, including 34 percent who used tai chi, yoga, or qi gong.

In a meta-analysis, which was conducted in Australia, the results of fifteen studies were reviewed. In thirteen of the studies, the use of tai chi was found to have a significant effect on the management of anxiety and depression. And at the University of Wisconsin-Milwaukee College of Nursing, experts looked at many studies of tai chi that were done between 1996 and 2004 among senior citizens. The authors concluded that tai chi is "low tech" and has "positive effects . . . due solely to its relaxing, meditative aspects."

YOGA

When something has been practiced for more than five thousand years, you assume it's got something positive going for it. Yoga is that something, and about 11 million Americans practice yoga and reap its health benefits. One of those health benefits is stress relief, and while not everyone who participates in yoga does so because they are anxious or stressed, stress reduction is a proven benefit of yoga.

There are many styles and forms of yoga, with some focused on relaxation and stress reduction while others are geared more toward developing strength, balance, and flexibility. That's not to say you can't improve your flexibility while reducing stress; you certainly can. However, if stress reduction is your main purpose, it's probably best to focus on a yoga style that promotes that goal, and then you can enjoy the added benefits as well.

Yoga typically involves three elements: physical poses (asanas or postures), controlled breathing, and in many cases, meditation. The intensity of each of these elements varies, depending on the style or form of yoga you choose.

Forms of Yoga

Although there are dozens of different forms of yoga, they all generally bring together physical and mental disciplines to achieve calm and balance of both body and mind. This goal is accomplished by utilizing various poses and controlled breathing, and often meditation as well.

Two specific types that are typically viewed as a good fit for relaxation and stress reduction are hatha yoga and Svaroopa yoga. Hatha yoga is one of the most common yogic styles and one of the easiest to learn. One advantage of hatha yoga is that it utilizes easier postures that are done at a slower pace than some other yoga styles. In addition, a key element of hatha yoga is controlled breathing, which can help improve oxygen delivery to the body and alleviate stress.

A more recently developed form of yoga is Svaroopa, which is a style of hatha yoga said to extend into the spine and help release the stress and tension people hold there and in their mind. Teachers of Svaroopa yoga often refer to the form as being based on the "core opening," which means the poses help release stress from the core of your being as well as support your spine, neck, and shoulders, where it often gathers.

"Svaroopa" is Sanskrit and means you get to know yourself at the deepest level of your being. The poses used in Svaroopa yoga also have a positive effect on your internal organs and glands, allowing your body to function in balance and harmony.

Svaroopa yoga is helpful for restoring mental and emotional balance, promoting inner calm, and improving one's self-awareness. All of this can be accomplished by positioning the body at precise angles and with the assistance of Svaroopa instructors, who are trained to help people make bodily adjustments that allow tension and stress to dissipate.

Svaroopa yoga makes use of lots of soft blankets as props, which participants use to support their back, knees, feet, and hips in various positions, and also cover the body to provide warmth and comfort. Sessions begin with shavasana (the corpse pose) in a modified form that allows the spine and body to settle gently into the floor and the mind to become calm. Shavasana is followed by a guided breathing session, and then various poses designed to release body tension. Instructors are helpful here, as they can assist you in finding the range of a position that best suits you.

Svaroopa yoga sessions end after forty-five minutes or so by returning to shavasana. There are beginning, continuing, and advanced levels of Svaroopa yoga. Certified Svaroopa yoga instructors must complete five hundred hours or more of training, including anatomy and physiology, meditation, and pose adjustments, before receiving certification. Some Svaroopa yoga teachers are certified as medical yoga therapists, so if you have a medical condition, be sure to look for an instructor who has received such training.

A type of yoga that is considered to be just beyond hatha yoga is called raja yoga, which is also known as classical yoga. While hatha yoga largely concentrates on poses and breathing, raja yoga focuses on poses to prepare the body for extended meditation. So if meditation is something you want to explore, raja yoga may be for you. (Also see "Deep Breathing Meditation for Stress.")

You may also find classes being offered in Iyengar yoga and Bikram yoga. Iyengar yoga focuses on body alignment and staying in certain poses for an extended period of time. Bikram yoga is done in an environment of high temperatures and high humidity. While it can help promote better breathing, circulation, and flexibility, it also can be unsafe for people who have certain medical conditions, such as heart disease or high blood pressure.

Along with stress reduction, yoga offers other benefits that complement its calming effect, such as:

- Improved flexibility, range of motion, and strength

- Better posture and balance

- Weight loss (can help women who tend to over-eat for emotional or stress-related reasons)

- Better management of health conditions such as depression, pain, insomnia, fatigue, and blood pressure

Before You Practice Yoga

Yoga is generally considered to be a safe activity for people of any age and ability level. However, be sure to check with your health-care provider if you have any health conditions that may present a risk, in which case you may need to find another stress-reduction activity or a different style of yoga. Some conditions to discuss with your health-care provider include balance problems, glaucoma (and other vision problems), uncontrolled high blood pressure, severe osteoporosis, pregnancy (but there are special yoga classes for pregnant women!), and joint replacements.

Yoga can be learned from a book or video, but it is recommended you attend at least a few classes so you can get help with poses and breathing techniques from a qualified instructor. Classes are typically offered by fitness centers and yoga studies, and also offered at community centers, schools, and churches. Before you sign up for a class, you should ask the following questions:

- Can you observe a class before signing up?

- Does the class focus on stress reduction, or is it geared toward other needs?

- How long has the instructor been practicing and teaching this form of yoga?

- Does the instructor have experience working with individuals who have health concerns?

(This is especially important if you have a health issue.)

• Do you need to bring your own yoga mat?

Yoga is a personal choice, and you may want to try several different forms before choosing the one that best suits you.

Yoga Studies

One study involved individuals with chronic diseases who were also overweight or obese. The eighty-six adult subjects participated in a program that included yoga postures, breathing exercises, stress management, group discussions, and individualized advice. The investigators noted that the participants experienced a reduction in cortisol levels and an increase in beta-endorphins (natural painkillers) in as little as ten days of practicing yoga.

At Duke University School of Medicine, investigators looked at the impact of yoga and mindfulness intervention on stress reduction among 239 employee volunteers. The volunteers were randomly assigned to a control group, yoga, or one of two mindfulness-based programs (which focus on moment-to-moment awareness). Both the yoga and mindfulness groups experienced significantly greater reductions in stress as well as improvements in sleep quality and heart rhythm than did volunteers in the control group. The authors concluded that "both mindfulness-based and therapeutic yoga programs may provide viable and effective interventions to target high stress levels."

BOTTOM LINE

Physical activity is an effective and healthful way to manage stress and promote your overall health. Be sure to schedule time to enjoy some type of physical exercise at least four to five times per week. If you are finding it difficult to "make the time" to exercise or you feel overwhelmed with other responsibilities, take a deep breath and remember DROP: delegate, reduce, organize, prioritize. You deserve to take care of yourself!

STEP 3

Relax and Clear the Mind

Are you ready for a vacation or at least a little time away from it all? It seemed like nearly every woman I spoke with about the stress in her life was ready for some time off, time away, or a chance to "chill out" alone. Yet their day-to-day responsibilities—their jobs, kids, partners, parents, friends, school and social obligations—were not granting them much respite, or at least that's how they perceived their situations. (Remember the discussion about perceived stress in chapter 2?) You may be familiar with these feelings, and if you are, then it's time to take ownership of your right to relax and clear your mind, at least for a while, each and every day. Because even if you think you don't have the time, you really do, and even more, you deserve it and it's essential for your overall well-being.

You can take minivacations from the demands and tension in your life without packing a suitcase, booking a cruise, or buying an airline ticket. And while you won't find yourself physically on a white endless beach, wooded mountaintop, or the streets of Paris, you will be there with the best companion you have: your mind. To that end, this chapter explains ways to relax and clear your mind and in the process, reduce, manage, or even banish stress, tension, and anxiety.

BREATHING THERAPY

You are already doing something that has been shown to be very effective in helping people relieve stress and to relax: breathing. However, you probably aren't breathing correctly. If this sounds strange (if you're thinking, "I know how to breathe . . . I've been doing it for X number of years with great success!"), the truth is, the majority of people don't breathe correctly, or at least in a way that promotes and supports health.

The way you breathe has an impact on every part of your body. When you breathe deeply and completely, you send life-supporting oxygen to all your cells while also reducing stress and tension. Once you learn how to breathe in a way that promotes relaxation, you can do breathing exercises anywhere, anytime—no equipment necessary! Breathing exercises also are an excellent technique to use along with yoga, guided visualization, and meditation to enhance your stress-reducing experience.

Breathing Exercises

There are many different forms of breathing exercises, and some are more complex than others. I will explain only the most basic—though still very effective—techniques so you can get started immediately. If you have never done any type of breathing exercises before, be sure to start with the first example, because it is the easiest one to learn. The other two examples are slightly more advanced, but you should be ready to try them once you are comfortable with the basic technique.

Basic Technique: Belly Breathing

- Sit or slightly recline in a comfortable position.

- Place one hand on your abdomen just below your rib cage and the other hand on your chest.

- Breathe in slowly and deeply through your nose and allow your abdomen to push your hand out. The hand on your chest should not move.

- Exhale slowly through your lips, as if you were whistling. You should feel the hand on your abdomen sink in, and you can help by pushing down on your belly to expel the air.

- Repeat this breathing exercise up to ten times. Relax and take your time with each breath.

Numbered Breathing

This is a variation of belly breathing.

- Place one hand on your abdomen and the other on your chest.

- Take a slow, deep breath through your nose and count to 4 as you send the air to your abdomen.

- Hold your breath and count from 1 to 7 silently.

- Slowly release your breath as you count from 1 to 8 to yourself. Don't rush! Try to release all your breath by the time you reach 8.

- Repeat this exercise up to eight times per session.

Rolled Breathing

Although you can do this type of breathing exercise sitting up, it is easier to learn it when lying on your back with your knees bent. This breathing technique can be very effective when you need to relax in a hurry.

- Place your left hand on your abdomen and your right hand on your chest.

- As you breathe in through your nose, focus on how your abdomen rises with each inhale and falls with each exhale. Also notice how the hand on your chest does not move. Repeat this breathing exercise eight to ten times.

- Now add the second step: inhale into your abdomen, and then continue to inhale into your upper chest. As you do, you should feel your left hand sink a little while your right hand (on your chest) rises, like a rolling motion.

- As you exhale, make a "whooshing" sound and release your stress and tension along with it.

- Repeat this sequence for about three to five minutes. Continue to focus on how your abdomen and chest rise and fall with each inhale and exhale.

Be sure to do this breathing exercise slowly. If you begin to feel dizzy, stop and wait until you feel stable, then get up slowly.

Lydia found that incorporating deep-breathing exercises into her daily routine really helps bring her stress level down. "I decided to make it part of my stress-reducing plan," she says, "and I also wanted to include my two kids in the breathing because it's good for them too, and it also helps me stick with my plan." Before her two children, six-year-old Simon and eight-year-old Madison, go to bed, they and Lydia practice deep breathing together.

"It's something we can do together, and it helps them wind down from their day and prepare them for sleep. Simultaneously, it helps me do the same thing. I also practice the rolling breathing during the day at work on my break and at lunch." Other elements of Lydia's stress-management plan include the addition of stress-reducing foods (see step 4) and walking five days a week before work. "I also intend to add yoga along with the deep breathing for both me and the kids as part of my plan," she says.

Deep Breathing Studies

Here are a few of the studies that have been done involving deep breathing and stress management. I chose studies that included different types of participants to illustrate how deep breathing can help reduce stress in a variety of situations.

- A study presented at a meeting of the American College of Chest Physicians in October 2012 reported on the effect of deep breathing and visualization on women and men with cardiovascular disease who were having difficulty with sleep and stress. The authors explored the impact of a ten-minute Tension Tamer on stress levels and sleep. A total of 334 volunteers (average age 56.6 years) were shown how to practice the Tension Tamer, which is a combination of deep breathing and visualization that individuals choose themselves. The technique was practiced at bedtime. Overall, use of the Tension Tamer technique improved perceived stress in 65 percent of the participants and also significantly improved sleep and level of fatigue.

- College students are typically under a lot of stress, and so they are a good population among which to perform stress studies. A study reported in the *Journal of Child and Adolescent Psychiatric Nursing* found that among college students under stress who also were being treated for depression, the common coping mechanisms they chose on their own included deep breathing, journaling, exercise, talking with friends (socializing), and listening to music. The authors also reported that "nonmedical methods of coping were often cited as more effective than medication therapy."

- Another high-stress group is patients who are battling serious disease, such as cancer. Therefore researchers explored the effects of deep breathing on a group of women with gynecologic cancer who were undergoing chemotherapy. Twelve women were assigned to a control group and eleven to a treatment group. Women in the treatment group were instructed on how to do abdominal breathing, thoracic breathing, and breathing while raising their arms. Analysis showed that women in the deep-breathing group experienced more relief from tension, anxiety, and fatigue than did women in the control group.

Thinking about adding deep breathing to your stress-reduction plan? That's great news, and you might want to take one additional step and incorporate the breathing with meditation, guided visualization, or yoga, or even include it before or after an exercise routine. Make your coffee break a breathing break, chill out while you're waiting for the bus, or make deep breathing a part of your bedtime routine, like Lydia and her children do!

GUIDED IMAGERY/VISUALIZATION

Do you like chocolate? Now close your eyes and imagine you are unwrapping a piece of your favorite chocolate candy. Do you hear the rustling of the paper? Now place the candy into your mouth. Can you taste it, feel the sweet texture of the chocolate on your tongue? Have I triggered a craving for chocolate? (Sorry!) If you were momentarily transported to a time and place where you "ate" chocolate, then you have an idea of what guided imagery can do.

Now take a moment to imagine you are walking along a clear mountain stream on a warm spring day while a light breeze, carrying the scent of wildflowers, brushes against your cheek. The bubbling of the stream is joined by the call of birds from high up in the trees, and the ground under your feet is covered with a layer of soft pine needles that cushion each step.

Feeling relaxed? You have just taken a trip courtesy of guided visualization, and without leaving your seat! A typical guided visualization session is longer than this brief introduction, although in as little as ten to twenty minutes, you can take a journey that allows you to shed your tension, stress, and negative emotions and enter a world of your choosing. When you choose to reenter the real world, you will hopefully be able to carry the good feelings with you for a while.

How Guided Imagery Works

Guided imagery is a technique that utilizes focused suggestions and thoughts to guide your imagination toward a balanced, relaxed state of being. The technique is based on the concept that the mind and body are connected, and therefore what affects one has an impact on the other. Experts know this concept to be true, as is illustrated by the fact that the majority of physical ailments are either caused by stress or have stress as a critical factor in their development and persistence.

Imagery is a basic language, but one without words. Individuals have the ability to recall images, events, sounds, smells, and tastes from the past, and it is this ability that helps makes guided imagery so powerful, especially when you combine these elements. When you imagined eating the piece of chocolate at the beginning of this chapter, you were asked to utilize not only a memory of eating chocolate, but also the sounds of opening the piece of candy, the texture of the chocolate on your tongue, and the sweet taste, which could then trigger a desire to grab a piece of chocolate! Combining various sensory elements can make the whole guided imagery experience more powerful and thus more beneficial.

Numerous clinical studies support the use of guided imagery for stress, depression, and other mental/emotional challenges, and it is frequently used as part of professional therapy sessions. Studies show guided imagery can reduce blood pressure, lower heart rate, and relieve muscle tension. People also use guided imagery to help them quit smoking, lose weight, and manage pain. Athletes frequently use guided imagery before competition, and public speakers and actors are known to practice it before stepping out on the stage or before a podium. All of these benefits are possible because imagery is a biological connection between the physical and the mental/emotional.

Olivia learned about guided imagery from her fifteen-year-old daughter's drama teacher. Sylvia had the lead role in *Romeo and Juliet* at her high school, and although a talented young lady, she was experiencing a lot of anxiety and stress, worrying she would forget her lines or make mistakes on stage. Her drama teacher, Ms. Martinelli, coached the teen on how to use guided imagery to help her overcome her fears. Sylvia learned how to imagine herself in different scenes performing with grace, confidence, and poise as she focused on the lights, the smell of the painted scenery, the feel of the floor under her feet, and the sound of applause.

When Olivia saw how guided imagery helped her daughter overcome her fears and allowed her to perform exceptionally well as Juliet, she realized she could learn to use guided imagery to deal with the stressors in her own life. "I was having some personality conflicts with one of my coworkers," says Olivia, who is a nurse at a large city hospital. "I worked with this person nearly every day, and the stress was putting me in a bad state of mind. Unfortunately, I then had a habit of letting my stress affect how I was dealing with patients, which was not a good thing."

With the help of several books and tapes on guided imagery, Olivia imagined several scenes with this individual and then she re-created them in her mind, imagining that the coworker was more giving, loving, and friendly. Olivia even came to realize that perhaps she was contributing to the animosity between them, and so the guided imagery sessions were also a lesson for her. "Over time, I found that the relationship I had with this coworker improved, and I also felt so much better about going to work."

Making Guided Imagery Work for You

You can practice guided imagery in the privacy of your home at a time of your choosing, or you can participate in a group session. If you have never tried a guided visualization before, you may find it helpful to participate in a group, or you may feel more comfortable learning about it from books, videos, or DVDs, which can provide you with a wide variety of scripts to follow for stress reduction (see the appendix).

Most people find they can master guided imagery after just a few sessions. Once you feel at ease with one or more different visualizations, try to practice several times a day. Suggested times are in bed before you get up in the morning (a great way to start your day!) and at night before going to sleep. Naturally, if an occasion arises during the day when guided imagery would help, go for it!

Feel free to combine guided imagery with other stress-management techniques. It's been shown that yoga, meditation, and progressive relaxation easily complement guided imagery. However, you may find other ways to incorporate this practice into your life, such as while exercising on a treadmill or stationary bike.

Here are some tips on how to do guided imagery.

- Find a place where you will not be disturbed for the duration of your "journey." You may choose to dim the lights.

- Wear comfortable clothing, take off your shoes, and find a cozy chair or bed. Some people prefer to get into a yoga pose.

- Close your eyes and take a few gentle, deep breaths as you begin your imaging journey.

- If you are using an audio script, follow the directions.

- If you are using your own mental script, continue your breathing exercise until you feel relaxed.

- Once you are relaxed, imagine the scene or situation you have chosen. It may be a beach, a café, a mountain meadow, a family gathering, or even an imaginary place where you feel safe and secure (like a grown-up's secret place or one you remember from childhood!).

- Experience the scene with all of your senses: smell the air, the food, the grass; sip the coffee or take a bite of an apple; hear the waves crash on the beach or the birds singing in the trees; hug your friends or splash in a stream.

- Identify your stress. Are you worried about making a speech? Fighting with your children over curfew? Are you experiencing chronic headaches or neck pain from stress?

- Prepare to send the stress on its way: pack it up in a suitcase and imagine putting it on an airplane all by itself. Send your stress up in a hot air balloon. Imagine your stress is carried away by the waves of the ocean or is overgrown by a massive bed of wildflowers in a field. It's up to you to imagine how to banish your stress.

- After you have sent your stress on its way, gradually exit your scene, saying good-bye to each of the elements of your imaginary location. Take a few deep breaths and picture yourself reentering your real environment.

- You are now ready to face the day!

Guided Visualization Studies

Although guided imagery is frequently used as a means of stress reduction by therapists and individuals on their own, few studies have examined its benefits. One of the studies was mentioned previously under "Deep Breathing," in which researchers evaluated the use of deep breathing and guided imagery in patients with cardiovascular disease, and the effects were positive.

In another study, researchers at the Department of Marriage and Family Therapy, University of Nevada–Las Vegas, examined the effect of cognitive behavioral therapy–based relaxation and guided visualization on stress and psychological symptoms. Individuals who were experiencing significant stress in their lives participated in three sessions, during which guided visualization scripts were used along with relaxation and breathing therapy techniques. After the sessions, the participants showed lower levels of stress and distress as well as reported fewer physical and psychological complaints.

The power of guided imagery can be seen when it is used to help alleviate physical symptoms. In fact, guided imagery can be especially helpful for cancer patients undergoing chemotherapy and who want to avoid stress and other side effects. One study of forty patients undergoing chemotherapy explored the impact of both music therapy and guided imagery on anxiety, nausea, and vomiting. When this combination of therapies was used, the patients had a significant decline in all three factors.

Pregnancy can be an especially stressful time for women, and any anxiety pregnant women experience during this time can have a negative impact on both their health and the health of the fetus. Therefore, finding ways to reduce and manage stress is especially important for both mother and child. A Canadian team reviewed eight studies (a total of 556 participants) that explored the impact of mind-body therapies on stress during pregnancy; five studies involved guided imagery. Overall, the reviewers found evidence that guided visualization was helpful in reducing anxiety at the early and middle stages of labor in one study, and was effective in reducing anxiety and depression postpartum in another study.

LAUGHTER

Quick, what's the funniest thing or moment you can remember, something that instantly brings a smile to your face or makes you want to laugh out loud? It could be a joke, something silly your dog or cat does, a scene from a TV show or movie, or a memory from your college party days. For me, I think of a scene from an *I Love Lucy* show when Lucy is working in a candy factory on an assembly line, and her boss speeds up the line, forcing Lucy to begin stuffing candy into her mouth. For some reason, that scene can still make me laugh.

It's not just an adage: laughter is good medicine, and there are even scientific studies to prove it (see "Laughter, Stress, and Science"). Although a good belly laugh or a case of the giggles isn't guaranteed to blow your blues away, it can provide both short-term and long-term benefits. Let's start with the short-term advantages. Laughter can:

- Flip the switch on your stress response, causing your blood pressure and heart rate to increase and then return to normal. The result is a calmer, relaxed feeling.

- Help your muscles relax and boost blood circulation, both of which can result in a calming effect.

- Boost the release of endorphins, the brain chemicals with natural mood-raising and pain-reducing properties.

- Improve the intake of oxygen, which in turn nurtures your lungs, heart, circulatory system, and muscles.

Now the long-term benefits. Laughter can:

- Improve your ability to cope with stressful or challenging situations.

- Relieve pain by increasing the release of endorphins, the body's natural painkillers.

- Enhance your immune system by releasing neuropeptides, chemicals that help fight stress.

"I'm not really a funny person," said Shelly when a group discussion among six women turned to the subject of laughter as the best medicine. "I laugh, but I don't find a lot of things to be funny." Shelly admits she tends to be a serious person, as well as a self-proclaimed cynic and "pretty stressed out." But after a few of her friends gently but persistently questioned her, she finally admitted she had a few favorite comics and was a "secret admirer" of the animated cat Garfield, who "just cracks me up."

Once the cat was out of the bag, so to speak, Shelly had found the beginning of her road to humor therapy to help with stress relief. She downloaded segments of routines from her favorite comedians to her tablet and has acquired a DVD collection of Garfield movies that she watches when she needs a break after a long day at work. Although Shelly admits she is still working on her overall stress-management plan, laughter therapy is a good start.

How can laughter de-stress your life? Identify the things that make you chuckle, laugh, and roll in the aisles. Then incorporate them into your day.

For example:

- Display pictures or sayings that make you smile. Put them in prominent places, such as at your work station, on the refrigerator, next to your bathroom mirror, on your dashboard, and on the back of your front door (so you'll see it when you leave the house).

- Make other people laugh. When you share a smile, it can be contagious. Share a funny video or picture via e-mail with a friend or family member (but don't do this during work hours!). Tuck a funny picture or saying into your kid's lunch or your partner's briefcase.

- Take a laughter break. Along with that cup of coffee or tea, check out a few short funny videos on the Internet. There's a nearly endless supply of funny short clips and videos you can see on Yahoo (lots of funny animal videos), YouTube, and other venues. Having trouble sleeping? Kids driving you crazy? Need a short break from paying bills? Watch a few humorous videos and you'll feel some of the stress liftoff your shoulders.

Laughter, Stress, and Science

Laughter can have a positive impact on your stress hormones, and scientists have proven it. At Loma Linda University in California, a research team studied the body's response to repetitive laughter and discovered that it has an effect that is similar to repetitive exercise. According to lead researcher Dr. Lee Berk, "studies have indicated that laughter can decrease cortisol and epinephrine (the hormones that regulate stress), help reduce blood vessel constriction and boost immune function."

Along with reducing stress, laughter also helps your entire cardiovascular system. At the University of Maryland Medical Center in Baltimore, a research team explored the effect of laughter on the inner blood vessel lining. The health of this lining is critical since your blood vessels transport life-supporting blood and nutrients throughout your body. When those vessels are compromised—and stress is one factor that can compromise them—then your health can suffer. In fact, studies show that mental stress and depression are associated with reduced endothelial (blood vessel lining) reactions.

However, the researchers found that "mirthful laughter" causes the release of chemicals called beta-endorphins, which trigger a series of events that benefit the blood vessels. Therefore, when you laugh, you help release stress and boost your cardiovascular system.

MEDITATION

If you visit the Web site for the Mayo Clinic concerning meditation, you are faced with an opening statement that says "Meditation can wipe away the day's stress, bringing with it inner peace." There was a time when you would not expect to see such a statement from a conventional medical establishment. Yet meditation is widely accepted as an effective, safe, and efficient way to cope with stress and, at the same time, effectively manage a wide variety of physical and emotional conditions. In addition, meditation doesn't cost you a dime, you can enjoy its benefits after just a few minutes, and you can do it in the privacy of your home or another location of your choosing, even while waiting in line at the grocery store. So what are you waiting for!

Benefits of Meditation

The benefits of meditation have been recognized and valued since ancient times. Originally meditation was used to help foster and deepen a person's relationship with spiritual and sacred forces in life. While this form of mind-body medicine is still used for this purpose, today it is more often valued as a way to help people relax and reduce stress and anxiety. Although a meditation session may last only a few minutes, its benefits can last for hours or even days. However, it is typically recommended that people who practice meditation do so on a daily basis to help support and nurture its benefits.

Remember Goldie Hawn, the award-winning and much-nominated movie actress and producer? In 2012, at age sixty-seven, she looked like she was toying with the half-century mark and had the vitality of people half her age. Her secret, she revealed during ah interview with *Prevention* magazine that same year, is meditation. Goldie apparently has been practicing meditation since the 1970s, and she has initiated a program that teaches children how to use meditation in the classroom to reduce stress and anxiety through mindfulness, a type of meditation (discussed below). According to Goldie, everyone should meditate and think of it "as an everyday task, like brushing your teeth."

Studies show that meditating for just three minutes a day five times a week can be as helpful as meditating for one twenty-minute session. So if you think you don't have the time to meditate, don't tell me you can't find just three minutes a day to spare!

These are some of the benefits of regular practice of meditation:

- Produces a sense of peace, harmony, and internal calm

- Helps you release stress, tension, and anxiety from your mind and body

- Helps you get a new perspective on the things in your life that are causing you stress and concern

- Provides you with a way to manage your stressors

- Increases self-awareness and self-confidence

- Helps you eliminate negative emotions

- Allows you to focus on the present rather than the past

- Helps you deal with health issues such as allergies, anxiety, depression, eating disorders, fatigue, high blood pressure, pain, and sleep problems

Types of Meditation

Meditation can be done in dozens of different ways, so what's the best way? The one that works best for you! If you are new to meditation, one way to decide which method fits your style is to read about several types of meditation and then try the ones that pique your interest. You can try them either alone, with a friend, or in a group setting. Many communities offer meditation classes or free introductory sessions at senior centers, fitness centers, churches, and community centers.

Since space does not permit me to list all the different types of meditation, here are some general categories.

- Mindfulness meditation. Also known as Vipassana, mindfulness meditation is a popular form in which individuals focus on an increased awareness and acceptance of the present moment, or "being in the moment." One way to do mindfulness meditation is to focus awareness on the flow of breath and nothing else. In mindfulness meditation, you detach from any encroaching thoughts or emotions, letting them pass by without making any judgments on them.

- Mantra meditation. If you are easily distracted, mantra meditation may be for you. In this type of meditation, you silently repeat a phrase, thought, word, or sound to yourself over and over again.

- Transcendental meditation (TM). This is a type of mantra meditation that became extremely popular during the 1960s and continues to be among the most commonly used forms of meditation in the world. The choice of mantra is said to be critical for transcendental meditation, and it should be chosen carefully so that it harmonizes with the individual. For this reason, it is best to get some training or participate in group TM sessions.

- Kundalini meditation. The term "Kundalini" is the name for the rising energy stream that is present in every person. The purpose of Kundalini meditation is to increase your awareness of this stream through concentration on the breath as it flows through each of the energy centers in the body.

- Heart rhythm meditation. This form of meditation focuses on both the breath (for balance) and the heartbeat (for energy). People who learn heart rhythm meditation are shown how to focus and direct their breath and their energy. The end result is a feeling of both control and sensitivity.

- Zazen meditation. Zazen is a general term for seated meditation. It is sometimes referred to as a minimal meditation and is said to be difficult to learn. Zazen meditation was original developed for monks, and it is often done along with focusing on a Buddhist scripture or spiritual question.

Other practices that incorporate meditation as part of their practice include guided imagery (which is considered to be a type of meditation), tai chi, yoga, and qi gong.

Is Meditation for You?

The only way you can answer this question is to explore various types of meditation and try them. Seek out introductory sessions in your community, watch videos or DVDs that explain different types of meditation, and talk to others who practice meditation.

According to Jeanne Ball, who has been practicing and teaching TM for more than twenty-five years, specializing in helping people with stress-related disorders, "I find that women these days do not have to be convinced that they need more rest and rejuvenation. But many do need assurance that it's okay to take the time."

Do you think you deserve to take the time to meditate? Only you can answer that question for yourself, but I did ask a friend who has made a fifteen-minute meditation a part of her daily life for years. She told me that her daily meditation is her lifeline and centering point. "That fifteen minutes is just for me—no kids, husband, dogs, work, parents, nothing, just me. I renew myself each and every time. I don't just deserve to meditate, I must meditate to stay focused and balanced. Often I do short meditations during the day as well, for just a few minutes. I can't recommend it enough."

SLEEP

This may sound like a silly question, but do you know how to sleep, I mean really sleep, so that you will wake up refreshed, stress-free, and full of vitality? Do you remember the last time you woke up in the morning and felt that good? If you are reading this section, chances are you haven't been sleeping well and are looking for some relief. It's also possible you're caught in a vicious cycle: not only may stress be a reason you can't sleep, but you also may be stressed about the fact that sleep is such a problem. Let's see how you can break the cycle.

Importance of Sleep

Sleep is one of the best remedies for stress, yet if worrying about your kids or your mother's health is keeping you up at night, you're not getting the sleep you need. Years of research on the importance of sleep have shown that sleep is essential for health in a variety of areas. For example:

- Memory and learning. You need sufficient sleep so your brain can properly catalog new information to memory.

- Mood. This probably comes as no surprise, since people who don't get enough sleep are often cranky, irritable, and moody.

- Energy. Lack of sufficient sleep can leave you unable to do the things you need to do and even result in fatigue.

- Weight and metabolism. People who suffer from chronic lack of sleep have a tendency to gain weight, and it's not always because they are raiding the refrigerator at midnight. Both hormones and how the body processes and stores carbohydrates are affected by a lack of sleep.

- Sickness. When you deprive your body of adequate sleep, the immune system begins to break down, including the activities of certain elements like killer cells that fight cancer. You also increase your risk of developing infections such as colds and flu.

- Heart health. Chronic sleep problems are associated with high stress-hormone levels, high blood pressure, and an increased risk of stroke, heart attack, irregular heartbeat, and heart failure.

- Personal safety. Lack of sleep at night makes you sleepy during the day, and you could fall asleep while driving or engaging in other activities and harm yourself and others. An inability to concentrate or remember information when you are overly tired may also result in accidents, making mistakes with medications and other serious decisions, or other safety issues.

- Longevity. People who regularly sleep less than six or seven hours per night have a greater risk of dying than do people who get more sleep.

How to Sleep

Getting enough refreshing sleep should be a Priority, so if you have to Delegate responsibilities, Organize your nighttime routine differently, or Reduce your intake of fluids at night, do it! Here are some tips on how to (1) reduce stress so you can prepare to get the refreshing sleep you need, and (2) get the sleep you need to help eliminate stress in your life:

- Sleeping well begins before you climb into bed, and by that I mean you need to get regular exercise. Since routine physical exercise is another recommended way to manage and banish stress, exercise offers two benefits! Do not exercise right before going to bed, however, because you will become energized from the physical activity, which will make falling asleep more difficult.

- Give yourself permission to get a good night's sleep. This may sound silly, but many women sabotage their sleep by believing they have to solve all of the day's problems before they can close their eyes. Wrong! The first step to getting restful sleep is to believe you deserve it. Once you do that, you can take steps to achieve it, and that should include the next tips.

- Develop a stress-reduction routine before settling down to sleep. Examples include doing tai chi, a short meditation, guided visualization, breathing exercises, self-hypnosis, hot bath, or progressive relaxation. Some women find that reading or listening to soothing music is relaxing. However, avoid picking up a thriller if you find you can't put it down!

- Establish a routine. Go to bed and get up at the same time every day, including weekends.

- Avoid filling up. Do not eat or drink anything substantial at least three hours before going to bed. A full stomach can cause gastrointestinal problems or prompt you to get up during the night. If you feel you need something to eat before going to bed, limit it to a small amount, such as four ounces of yogurt or a small apple. Also limit liquids to avoid having to get up to go to the bathroom during the night.

- Create a sleep-friendly environment. Is your sleeping space conducive to a restful, stress-free night of sleep? That includes comfortable temperature, bedclothes, pillow, and mattress. How about sound? Some people like low background sound like low-playing classical music or the sound of water falling. Other people need silence to sleep well. If there are environmental sounds that disturb your sleep, get earplugs. How about light? Darkness is best for sleep, as exposure to light stimulates an area of the brain called the hypothalamus, which in turn triggers the release of the stress hormone cortisol. Darkness stimulates the pineal gland to produce melatonin, which helps you feel drowsy. Levels of melatonin remain elevated for about twelve hours during the night and return to barely detectable levels during the day. It's best to keep your sleeping environment as dark as possible, although you may feel more secure with a small, strategically placed night-light in case you need to get up during the night, or keep a small flashlight on your nightstand.

- Avoid stimulation. Except for sex (I'm not trying to put a crimp in your sex life!), your bed should be for sleeping. Watching TV, playing video games, or working on your laptop while in bed can make it difficult to fall asleep. Another stimulant to avoid before bedtime is caffeine, which is found in coffee, tea, chocolate, and some medications. It can take four or more hours for caffeine to be eliminated from your body, so be sure to avoid caffeinated products for at least that long before bedtime.

- Don't look at the clock. If you wake up during the night and see that it's "only" two A.M. you may become stressed or anxious. If you have an alarm clock, turn the face away so you don't see it during the night.

If falling asleep and staying asleep are a chronic problem, you should also consider the possibility you have a sleep disorder. If you have a sleep partner, ask him or her if you ever stop breathing during the night (sleep apnea) or if you snore. Many people have an undiagnosed sleep disorder and are suffering needlessly when something can be done about it.

If you would like some extra, natural help with sleep, then you might consider taking the natural hormone melatonin. As women get older, their melatonin production tends to decline, while their nighttime cortisol levels can be more than thirty times higher than when they were just a few decades younger. Therefore, a melatonin supplement may help boost melatonin production and improve your natural sleep cycle (see step 4, "Nourish and Replenish").

STEP 4

Nourish and Replenish

How many times have you found yourself mindlessly eating potato chips from a bag, scooping ice cream from a quart container with a teaspoon, or reaching again and again for a handful of nuts or little pieces of chocolate? More times than you'd like to admit? You're not alone; you are a member of the comfort eaters club, and you share this stress-eating habit with perhaps millions of other women (and men).

It's no secret that many people find comfort in food, but it's also generally accepted that most people wouldn't name broccoli, apples, lettuce, and grapes on their top ten list of foods they turn to when they're feeling stressed or in need of comfort. Why? Because foods that typically fall into the comfort-food kettle have qualities—namely, fat and sugar—that work on brain chemicals and produce a feeling of calm, at least temporarily. Unfortunately, broccoli doesn't have the same effect, even though it is a much more nutritious choice overall.

Yet you can also use healthful, delicious foods to nourish and replenish your body and mind. There are many tasty foods that can help regulate and even lower levels of the stress hormone cortisol. In addition, there are numerous herbs and other natural substances that can support efforts to reduce stress and bring calm, harmony, and peace to your body, mind, and spirit.

The purpose of this chapter is to introduce you to foods and natural supplements, including herbal and homeopathic remedies and nutrients, that you can incorporate into your daily life to reduce and manage your stress, nurture your overall health, and replenish your reservoirs.

Will changing your diet and adding stress-reducing natural supplements to your life completely overhaul your body and leave you entirely stress-free? That would be great, but likely not. However, what changing your diet can do, if you adopt DROP and incorporate other stress-reduction techniques, is greatly improve the quality of your life and allow you to feel nourished and replenished every single day and with every meal. And that would be a pretty good feeling, don't you think?

FOODS AND STRESS

In chapter 2, I discussed how women who experience stress frequently seek comfort in sugary, salty, high-carb, high-fat foods. That's because chronic, prolonged exposure to the stress hormone cortisol throws the body's metabolism into a tizzy, triggering cravings for foods that are not healthful. The chocolate and other high-carbohydrate foods that you crave boost your levels of the hormone serotonin, which provides a calming effect. Research also suggests that a combination of sugar and fat (sounds like chocolate!) can make you feel more peaceful.

This phenomenon has been shown in rats. When investigators from the University of California at San Francisco exposed rats to a high-stress environment, they discovered that the animals who were highly stressed wanted to eat fat and sugar, and when they did, their brains made fewer stress hormones. While one part of this phenomenon may sound like a good thing, the negative side is that eating fat and sugar is not healthful for a variety of reasons, including a greater risk of diabetes, obesity, heart disease, and a wide range of cancers.

To add insult to injury, you would think being stressed would cause you to burn calories, but instead stress makes your body metabolize fewer calories, and then cortisol can lower the body's ability to release fat from storage so you can burn it. And because stress hormones cause fat to accumulate in the abdominal area, many women end up with belly fat that is difficult to lose.

Here are a few tips to help fight stress. Be prepared to institute the "Reduce" part of DROP!

- Limit or eliminate caffeine from your diet. I know this can be a difficult step for some women, but here's why it's important. Caffeine causes a rise in cortisol, as much as 30 percent in just one hour, and this effect can last most of the day. If eliminating caffeine seems like too drastic a move, do it slowly. Gradually switch to decaffeinated coffee, incorporate tea into your routine, and try herbal (no caffeine) teas.

- Avoid sugars. Again, this can be a challenge, depending on how much sugar you are used to eating regularly in your current diet. Refined carbohydrates like simple sugars provoke drastic increases in insulin production and cause blood sugar levels to rise, which stresses the adrenal glands and their ability to regulate the level of stress hormones in the body. Refined sugar also stimulates the release of the brain chemical called dopamine, which makes you feel pleasure and also makes you want more of the same. A study from 2010 reported that sugar causes the release of endorphins in the brains of some people in a way that is very much like how cocaine and similar drugs release endorphins. If you are thinking, "All this talk about refined sugar makes it sound like a drug addiction," you're right. Morphine, heroin, and sugar all work on the same trigger points, or receptors, in the brain. To help wean yourself off sugar, gradually reduce the sugary foods in your diet and replace them with naturally sweet foods, such as whole fruits. Many foods contain hidden sugar, so be sure to read labels carefully. (Also see "The Unsweet Side of Sugar and Stress.")

- Stay clear of trans fats. Fortunately, it's becoming easier to avoid these dangerous synthetic fats since food manufacturers have been required to list the trans fat content on their labels. However, trans fats still lurk in many cakes, cookies, pies, crackers, and other baked goods, as well as in some frozen and prepared foods such as dinners, salad dressings, puddings, and breads. Therefore, make sure you read labels carefully and look for telltale signs of trans fats, such as the terms "hydrogenated oil," "partially hydrogenated oil," or "margarine." Food labels also list the amount of trans fat that may be found in the product. Trans fats not only jeopardize heart health, they also compromise the immune system, which places more stress on the body.

- Watch your alcohol use. Alcohol is a significant source of sugars, a fact that is easy to forget. While surveying women during the writing of this book, I often heard from them that one way they coped with stress was "a glass or two of wine," or "a few drinks." Moderate alcohol consumption for women is considered to be one drink per day (which translates into five ounces of wine, twelve ounces of beer, or one ounce of whiskey). Excessive alcohol use compromises the function of the adrenal glands, which are a protective barrier against stress.

- Hydrate. If you allow yourself to become dehydrated, you trigger a rise in cortisol levels and also stress your body. A simple suggestion is to keep a container of pure water with you throughout the day and by your bedside (add a slice of lemon to make it more palatable!).

If you make some minor modifications to your diet, you may reduce the effects of stress on your body and your emotional health. I'm not promising that making changes to your diet will have a dramatic effect on how you relate to stress and anxiety, but nutritional modifications can have a cumulative positive impact not only on your stress response but on your overall health, and that in turn cycles back to supporting and nurturing your body, mind, and spirit.

For example, did you know that foods that are low on the glycemic scale and high in protein can help lower cortisol levels? Cortisol causes your blood sugar levels to rise, which in turn results in acidic blood and serious health conditions such as cancer, diabetes, excessive abdominal fat, and heart disease. Therefore, it makes sense to focus on foods with a low glycemic index (which are also naturally low in sugar) and high in protein.

Okay, so what are the best foods you can eat to both help reduce stress and make you feel calmer? Fortunately, there are many foods that fall into this category, and they aren't all rice cakes and celery! Here are some suggestions of foods to include in a low-stress diet:

- Apricots (dried), which are high in magnesium, a mineral that helps relax tense muscles.

- Avocados, fruits that are high in monounsaturated fats and potassium and thus help lower blood pressure. Avocados have more potassium than bananas (which can also help bring your blood pressure down, so include them as well).

- Beans, such as black beans, chickpeas, kidney, navy, and pinto beans.

- Chia seeds. They can be ground and added to smoothies and sprinkled on salads, vegetables, and soups.

- Chicken and turkey. While both forms of fowl have stress-reducing properties, turkey is the one with the amino acid called L-tryptophan, which stimulates the release of the brain chemical serotonin. This chemical is associated with a positive mood, a feeling of relaxation and even tiredness. (Do you feel sleepy after eating turkey on Thanksgiving?)

- Eggs. You can skip the yolks if dietary cholesterol is a problem for you.

- Fish. Especially cold-water fatty fish such as salmon, herring, tuna, and sardines.

- Flaxseeds. Use like chia seeds.

- Green, leafy vegetables such as arugula, collards, kale, mustard greens, red leaf lettuce, spinach, and turnip greens.

- Gluten-free grains, such as amaranth, buckwheat, brown rice, millet, quinoa (these are important because high-gluten foods such as those containing wheat can cause inflammation, which then leads to secretion of cortisol).

- Lentils, which are also a great source of protein and fiber.

- Olive oil (in moderation).

- Quinoa, a nutritious grainlike food that is a complete protein as well as a great source of stress-reducing B vitamins.

- Seeds, including pumpkin, sesame, and sunflower seeds, which are great sources of vitamin E.

- Sweet potatoes, which are not only a supernutritious food, but also have stress-reducing abilities since they offer both carbohydrates and a sweet taste to satisfy the comfort-food urge. In addition, they are chock-full of fiber and vitamins, including beta-carotene.

- Walnuts (which are high in omega-3 fatty acids), almonds, and pistachios. These nuts are great sources of B and E vitamins, which support the immune system and lower blood pressure (walnuts and pistachios).

- Winter squash, such as acorn, butternut, and spaghetti.

- Yogurt, either nonfat or low-fat dairy or soy, to which you can add fresh fruits and nuts.

Also include lots of foods that are high in vitamin C. That's because stress, and especially chronic stress, depletes the body's supplies of vitamin C. Since vitamin C is a water-soluble vitamin, it is eliminated continuously from the body in urine, so it is important to keep replenishing your reserves. The foods that are great for providing vitamin C include the following:

- Bell peppers (especially red, yellow, and orange peppers). These are a super source of vitamin C, with the yellow bells topping the list. Since they are so versatile, be sure to add them to as many recipes as you can to reap the most from these veggies.

- Berries. Enjoy blackberries, blueberries, cranberries, huckleberries, raspberries, and strawberries. It's strawberries that top the berry list for vitamin C, providing more than 163 percent of daily value per one-cup serving. However, you can boost the vitamin C power of your berries by combining them, so don't let your strawberries sit in the bowl alone!

- Cantaloupe and other melons.

- Citrus. Choose from grapefruit, clementines, tangerines, oranges, lemons, limes. All the citrus fruits, as natural, unsweetened juices as well as whole fruits, are excellent sources of vitamin C. The peels of citrus (zest) also provide vitamin C, and if you can add some grated zest to salads, smoothies, sandwiches, and soups, you'll be getting an extra boost of vitamin C.

- Cruciferous vegetables. Broccoli, Brussel sprouts, and cauliflower top the list of the cruciferous veggies that provide large amounts of vitamin C. These vegetables also have cancer-fighting benefits, so they are especially healthful.

- Dark green, leafy vegetables. Raw kale tops the list in this category, although it may be a bit challenging to eat. Even if you cook it lightly, you can still reap the rewards. Mustard greens are a close second, and they are delicious when stir-fried lightly with fresh garlic and onion. Other dark green veggies in this category include garden cress, spinach, collard greens, and beet greens.

- Guava. Depending on the variety of guava, you can get more than 600 percent of your recommended daily value from a single guava.

- Herbs. Thyme and parsley provide the most vitamin C of the common herbs, with basil following as a close third. Be sure to add them either fresh or dried as often as you can to your meals.

- Hot chili peppers (both red and green). If you can handle the heat, you'll be getting a great shot of vitamin C, because hot chili peppers rank number one on the scale of vitamin C for vegetables and fruits. Add just a small amount of chopped chili peppers to soups, stews, casseroles, and sandwiches.

- Kiwi. These small green or golden fruits are frequently forgotten, but they are an excellent source of vitamin C, kicking in nearly 300 percent of the recommended daily value for each cup. Although they are great to eat alone, they are a tasty addition to hot and cold cereals, assorted fruit bowls, swirled in a smoothie, or dipped in nonfat yogurt.

- Papayas. This tropical fruit provides lots of vitamin C as well as folate and vitamin A.

Diana's Story

Diana is a forty-six-year-old manager of a large clothing outlet store in Casa Grande, Arizona. She had been suffering with chronic headaches for years, and all of her attempts to quell the pain with a variety of over-the-counter medications in increasing doses had not helped. While experiencing one of her headaches at work one day a few months before Christmas, her good friend Sandy dropped in and asked Diana how she felt.

"Well, I'm trying to brace myself for the holidays," she said. "And if I keep having these headaches, it's going to be a real challenge. I can't seem to get rid of them." Sandy reached into her purse, pulled out a piece of paper, and jotted down a name and phone number.

"I hope you don't mind my saying this, but you looked so stressed all the time, and you've been having these headaches for far too long. My sister has a naturopath who helped her get rid of her headaches, and all without pills. Here's her name and number. Think about it, okay?"

Diana accepted the piece of paper from her friend, but it was another week before she made the call. Her introductory visit with the doctor lasted nearly an hour, but as she said later, it was the best hour she had spent in a long time.

"She asked me the normal questions about my health history and my family's history, but then she really delved into my diet, sleep habits, how I spent my leisure time, my exercise habits, and social and spiritual networks. She recommended I make some lifestyle changes to address the stressors in my life, which she believed were at the core of my chronic headaches. She emphasized dietary changes and gave me a list of recommended foods, and then she asked me to write down my plan of action and to come back in two weeks with plan in hand and how I was implementing it.

"When I questioned her about why changing my diet was so important, she just laughed and asked me if I put water in my gas tank or the recommended fuel. She said, 'How do you expect your body to function properly if you fill it with the wrong fuel? When you give your body inferior food or the wrong food, the body becomes stressed and struggles, like your car would sputter and not go.' So, I looked at the recommended food list and started to make some changes in my eating habits, including eliminating wheat and caffeine and adding lots of fresh fruits and vegetables."

While dietary changes were not the only items on Diana's action plan (she also added meditation and a walking program four days a week), she said that after just one month, her headaches had subsided significantly, and she felt better overall. "I have more energy and I feel good about taking care of myself. I know these changes are the reason for the difference, and the change in my diet has really helped turn my life around."

How to Avoid Junk Food

Your boss yelled at you all day. Your kids won't stop fighting. You're overdrawn at the bank . . . again. You're worried about your presentation to the entire financial committee tomorrow. Maybe there's nothing in particular that has you feeling stressed, but the bottom line is, you just have a craving for junk food. That pint of ice cream or bag of pork rinds is familiar, comfortable, and it doesn't talk back—or does it? Comfort food does talk back in the form of indigestion, feelings of guilt ("Did I really eat that entire bag of chips?"), weight gain, and as more fuel for the cycle of stress. So what can you do to help you handle cravings for junk food?

✓ Don't buy junk food or have it in the house. This is an obvious tip, but it can be a challenging one for women to follow, especially those who have children or a partner who doesn't want to buy into the "no comfort or junk food" plan. If that's the case, then you may have to establish a "comfort food" zone where other family members keep their goodies, unless you can control your cravings by having just one cookie instead of a handful or one serving of potato chips instead of the entire bag.

✓ Don't get hungry. If you forget to eat or you consciously avoid meals, you will likely have a tendency to overeat or eat comfort foods when you finally do eat. The safest and healthiest approach is to consume small meals or healthy snacks throughout the day to help keep your sugar and energy levels balanced, as well as your mood and stress levels.

✓ Eat consciously. If you practice meditation, it can actually help you learn to eat mindfully. In fact, you can do a type of meditation with food (see "How to Meditate with Food"). This can be a highly effective way to curb stress-induced eating if you practice it enough! You can get some meditation tips in step 3.

✓ Write it down. Keep a journal or diary of your food cravings, when you experience them, what you are feeling at the time, which foods you crave, and how much (if any) of the food you eat each time a craving strikes, you should see a behavior pattern. Once you are more aware of your emotions and the situations that trigger your cravings, you will be better equipped to take steps to manage them. Knowledge is power!

✓ Move! Whenever you feel a food craving coming on, get moving. Take a brisk walk, take the dog out, practice tai chi or yoga, rake leaves, clean out the garage, or do stretching exercises.

✓ Take a minvacation. When you get the urge to eat a large take-out portion of French fries or a pint of ice cream, take a vacation. Use of guided imagery can be helpful whenever you want to reach for junk food. Treat yourself to a minivacation in your head and leave the greasy or sugary foods behind.

✓ Keep lower-calorie foods readily available. This option works best if you like the lower-calorie foods. So if you really dislike the taste of sugar-free ice cream and you make yourself eat it, you may end up raising your stress level out of frustration. Even artificial sweeteners are stressful on the body. In fact, use of artificial sweeteners can actually make you crave more sweets. Some studies have evaluated the replacement of sugar-sweetened beverages with those sweetened with artificial sweeteners, and the investigators have not seen any difference in weight loss. Why? The answer is in the next item!

✓ Limit or avoid artificial sweeteners. One reason is that artificial sugars increase a person's craving for sugar. Some experts believe the body may not only recognize the sweetness of artificial sugars, but also expect the calories. However, since the calories are not there, then the body "craves" them, so you end up eating more and more of the food. Studies in rats have explored this very phenomenon, and scientists found that rats who were fed diets with artificial sweeteners consumed more calories all day than the animals who were fed meals that contained sugar. Artificial sweeteners may trigger the appetite centers of the brain to increase your cravings for more sweetness. Another possibility is that because artificial sweeteners are many times sweeter than refined sugar, the bodies of people who switch to artificial sweeteners become trained to expect the much greater sweetness associated with artificial sweeteners. Since consuming artificial sweeteners makes the body expect sweeter tastes, it does not have an opportunity to become familiar with the less-sweet taste of refined sugar.

THE UNSWEET SIDE OF SUGAR AND STRESS (AND HOW TO FIGHT IT)

You may love your sweets and especially crave chocolate, but unless you are able to limit your intake to very small amounts, you may feel the unsweet side of sugar, which can be especially damaging to women who eat too much of this refined "food." This also includes all simple carbs such as white bread and white pasta. One reason is that eating sugary and simple carb foods promotes the overgrowth of bacteria such as candida, which can lead to a systemic yeast infection known as candidiasis. This syndrome is associated with symptoms that can affect the entire body, making your life stressful and miserable. Some of those symptoms include fatigue, oral thrush, weakness, diarrhea, vaginitis, acne, irritable bowel syndrome, dizziness, pain, chronic headache, insomnia, irritability, memory problems, confusion, and depression.

Here are some other unsweet ways sugar can stress your body:

- Suppresses the immune system, making you susceptible to infections besides candidiasis, such as the common cold, flu, and bronchitis

- Promotes the development of some cancers

- Contributes to weight gain and obesity

- Sets up the body for the development of insulin intolerance and diabetes

- Upsets the balance of good cholesterol and bad cholesterol

While some women are able to eat a small amount of sugar and be satisfied, others climb aboard the sugar train and can't seem to get off once their brain chemicals are set in motion to crave this legal addiction. You know which category you are in, so plan accordingly. That said, here are some tips to fight your cravings for sugar:

- **Wake up with protein.** Put down that sugar doughnut, bagel, croissant, or bowl of cereal and pick up some protein. Starting your day with protein can help curb sugar cravings throughout the day. You might choose a nonfat yogurt smoothie with fresh fruit, an egg-white omelet with mushrooms, or an apple stuffed with almond butter.

- **Treat yourself.** If you don't want to forgo sweets entirely (and I know that's a difficult road to take!), then use them as rewards or treats for special occasions. When you do choose sweets, select those with less or no refined sugars. Examples include dark chocolate or items made with honey, natural fruit juices, molasses, agave syrup, or pure maple syrup. Another option you can use in moderation is xylitol, which is as sweet as refined sugar but has about 40 percent fewer calories and is about 75 percent lower in carbohydrates. Unlike refined sugar, xylitol is metabolized slowly in the body. It does not support candidiasis, nor does it have the impact on insulin that sugar has. The natural herb stevia, available in several convenient forms, is another option.

- **Don't kick yourself!** If you fall off the sugar-free wagon, don't stress out over it. Instead, choose to do something that rewards you for recognizing you slipped, like watching humorous movies or videos on the Internet, practicing a guided imagery session, or doing yoga. Then treat your body to a minidetox: eight ounces of hot water and the juice of half a lemon. When you get up the next morning, start your day with the same lemony beverage. It's a new day, so shake off the feelings of guilt and stress and decide to do better.

- **Limit alcohol intake.** The body metabolizes alcohol as pure sugar, and it can stimulate you to overeat and to choose sugary or refined foods. Substitute sparkling water with lemon or lime or a splash of unsweetened cranberry juice instead of wine, beer, or liquor.

- **Stop sugar cravings naturally.** Some natural supplements can help curb sugar cravings. You might try 500 mg to 1,000 mg of glutamine, which is an essential amino acid the body makes from glutamic acid, another amino acid. An interesting fact about glutamine is that a body under stress can be deficient in glutamine, which is why this supplement is frequently used to help boost the immune system. To curb sugar cravings, open up a glutamine capsule, place the contents under your tongue, and drink a few ounces of water. The suggested dose is 500 mg three to four times daily. Or you might try alpha-lipoic acid (100 mg twice daily), chromium (200 to 600 micrograms daily), N-acetycysteine (NAC; 600 to 1,200 mg twice daily), or the essential amino acid DL-phenylalanine (500 mg once daily, increasing to 1,500 mg daily as needed). Consult a healthcare provider before using these supplements.

HOW TO MEDITATE WITH FOOD

Choose a food you enjoy—a big juicy strawberry or perhaps a bite-sized piece of chocolate. (Ice cream doesn't work well with this meditation!)

Cut the portion in half and place it in your mouth.

Close your eyes and chew the morsel slowly while you focus on how it feels in your mouth, its sweetness, its texture, even its smell. Thoroughly chew the morsel until it has nearly dissolved in your mouth, then swallow it.

continued

Recall any pleasurable memories you may have about this particular food. Chocolate may remind you of baking chocolate chip cookies with your grandmother. Strawberries may make you think of summer strawberry festivals or picnics.

Pause for at least one minute after swallowing the food and savor its lingering taste in your mouth and your memory.

Then place the other half of the portion in your mouth and repeat the meditation.

NATURAL REMEDIES FOR STRESS CONTROL

A variety of natural supplements can help manage stress, support a sense of calm and peace, and help balance the body's response to stressors. Let's look at three categories of these natural remedies: natural nutrients (e.g., vitamins, minerals, and other similar substances, including the natural hormone melatonin), adaptogen herbs, and other herbs.

Natural Nutrients

Perhaps the most common nutrient or group of nutrients associated with stress reduction is the B family of vitamins. In fact, B vitamins are often sold as or referred to as stress-reducing vitamins and are available as a B-complex. Although there are eight main B vitamins and all have some role in stress, the ones most associated with stress reduction are the following:

- Thiamine (B_1). Essential for transforming sugar into energy, maintaining balanced nervous system function, and improving mental concentration.

- Niacin (B_3). The body makes niacin from the amino acid L-tryptophan. If you have low niacin levels, you are less able to handle stress and can experience irritability and depression.

- Pyridoxine (B_6). This B vitamin assists the body in manufacturing serotonin and other neurotransmitters involved in helping the body cope with stress, anxiety, and depression.

- Folic acid (B_9). The body can't make folic acid on its own, so if you allow your folic acid levels to decline, you may experience depression which in turn may lead to higher levels of stress.

- Cyanocobalamin (B_{12}). This B vitamin is the brains of the complex because the brain is the organ that requires this nutrient for healthy neurological function and memory. You also need vitamin B_{12} for the production of melatonin (the hormone that helps you sleep) and serotonin (a hormone involved in mood).

The B vitamins are a family and they work synergistically and so if you take B vitamins, it's advisable to take the B-complex, which in addition to the above B vitamins also includes B_2 (riboflavin), B_5 (pantothenic acid), B_7 (biotin), and choline, the newest addition to the B vitamin family and one without a number! B vitamins are water-soluble, which means you need to replenish your body's supply daily because you lose them in your urine. Many foods are an excellent source of one or two

B vitamins, but the B vitamins are widely distributed in many foods at varying levels. Foods that have more of the B vitamins than others include legumes (e.g., lentils, split peas, beans), green leafy vegetables, and fortified cereals. Other very good sources include yogurt, avocados, and seafood.

Several other natural substances may help reduce the impact of stress on the body. If you believe you are not getting a sufficient amount of these nutrients, you should consider taking a supplement (but consult your healthcare provider first). Here's a brief rundown of these nutrients and how they work:

- **Calcium and magnesium.** You probably know calcium is essential for strong bones, but it also has a role in stress. In fact, both calcium and another mineral, magnesium, need to be properly balanced for you to be able to recover from stress. An imbalance between calcium and magnesium also can be a source of stress. Here's how it works: when you experience stress, calcium enters your cells (say, muscle cells) and causes levels of the mineral inside the cells to rise. Magnesium then helps push the calcium out, which allows the muscle cells to relax. But if your calcium and magnesium levels are not balanced, calcium can continue to enter the cells and not allow them to relax. Magnesium also has an ability to prevent the nervous system from becoming overexcited, which is one reason why this mineral assists in maintaining a healthy blood pressure. The recommended daily allowance of calcium for women is 1,000 mg up to age fifty and then 1,200 mg thereafter, and for magnesium the RDA is 310 to 320 mg. Many women do not get enough magnesium, and low levels can be caused by emotional stress, use of certain drugs (e.g., oral contraceptives, diuretics, antibiotics), and too much calcium. Among the richest sources of magnesium are pumpkin seeds, dark green leafy vegetables, soybeans, sesame seeds, halibut, cashews, and almonds. Calcium sources include dark green leafy vegetables, dairy (low-fat and nonfat preferred), sardines (with bones), almonds, soybeans, sesame seeds, and flax seeds.

- **Chromium.** This mineral has already been mentioned as one that may suppress sugar cravings, but it also may help in reducing the effects of stress on the body. Low levels of chromium may reduce your body's production of a hormone called DHEA (dehydroepiandrosterone), which is produced by the adrenal glands, considered to be an antiaging hormone, and a hormone that modulates the stress response. Keeping your chromium at a healthy level can maintain DHEA as well and help you better cope with stress. Chromium supplements are available, and the recommended forms are GTE chromium and chromium picolinate. Suggested doses are 100 to 200 micrograms daily. The best dietary sources include brewer's yeast, cereals, dried fruit, molasses, and nuts.

- **Vitamin C.** I already mentioned vitamin C in the section on foods for stress. It is worth emphasizing that if you don't get enough vitamin C daily (the RDA is only 75 mg; 110 mg if you smoke), then you should consider taking a supplement. However, a mere six ounces of orange juice exceeds a

woman's RDA and half a grapefruit puts you
more than halfway there.

- **Zinc.** This mineral can help with stress in two
  ways: it's a potent antioxidant that can boost your
  immune system (which becomes compromised
  when you're experiencing chronic stress) and thus
  fight off infection, and it can also improve your
  ability to cope with stress. A woman's RDA for
  zinc is 30 mg, and the richest food sources are
  oysters, toasted wheat germ (untoasted wheat
  germ also has zinc, but about 25 percent less),
  roasted pumpkin and squash seeds (you can make
  your own in the oven), crab, and unsweetened
  baking chocolate and cocoa powder.

Adaptogen Herbs

Some herbs have properties that help nurture and support
the body's response to stress. These herbal remedies are
sometimes called tonics, and more accurately called
adaptogens. An adaptogen is an herb or other substance
that assists the body in adapting to stress by increasing its
ability to resist stressors while also helping it maintain
balance. Experts believe adaptogens work by increasing
the ability of the body's cells to make and use fuel more
efficiently. Adaptogen herbs are often referred to as the
great equalizers.

Another characteristic of adaptogen herbs is that they
work synergistically; that is, to get the most punch you
should take several adaptogens in a formula. In this sense,
more is better when it comes to taking adaptogen herbs,
but you still should not take megadoses of any of these
herbs: the rule with adaptogen herbs is combination in
moderation.

That said, let's look at some of the adaptogen herbs that have demonstrated an ability to balance the body's response to stress.

Rhodiola

Rhodiola rosea has a long reputation as an adaptogen herb. Part of that reputation is associated with the fact that the plant grows in some of the most stressful areas of the world: the Arctic, Siberia, the Rocky Mountains, the Alps, Pyrenees, and Iceland. This herb is inherently hardy!

Rhodiola appears to have an impact on levels of monoamine neurotransmitters, which include serotonin, dopamine, and melatonin, among others that have an effect on the brain. This could explain why Russians have claimed for centuries that rhodiola seems to help balance mood and relieve depression and even schizophrenia. Rhodiola also has been credited with aiding sleep, fatigue, irritability, high blood pressure, and poor appetite, all of which are signs of stress.

Scientific studies support the claims that rhodiola helps relieve stress. For example, a 2012 British study looked at the therapeutic effects of rhodiola extract in 101 individuals who had life-stress symptoms. All of the participants received 200 mg of rhodiola twice daily for four weeks, and they all completed seven questionnaires regarding their stress symptoms. The participants experienced an improvement in symptoms in as few as three days after starting treatment, and improvements continued throughout the study. None of the subjects reported serious side effects, and overall the 200 mg twice-daily dose proved to be safe and effective.

In a double-blind study, sixty women and men who were suffering with stress-related fatigue took either 576 mg of rhodiola extract daily or placebo. Both before and after the twenty-eight days of treatment, the participants completed questionnaires regarding symptoms, quality of life, depression, and attention, and they also had their saliva analyzed for cortisol levels. A comparison of all test results at the end of the study revealed that regular use of rhodiola "exerts an anti-fatigue effect that increases mental performance, particularly the ability to concentrate, and decreases cortisol response to awakening stress in burnout patients with fatigue syndrome." In other words, rhodiola appears to be an effective natural approach to managing stress.

Some people may experience side effects with rhodiola, including an increase in blood pressure. Because rhodiola may also cause thinning of the blood, you should consult your health-care provider if you are taking aspirin, warfarin, or other drugs or supplements such as vitamin E or garlic. If you are pregnant or breastfeeding, talk to your doctor before starting rhodiola.

Asian Ginseng

Few herbs have been as widely studied or as commonly used as Asian (or Korean) ginseng (*Panax ginseng*), which is not the same as American ginseng or Siberian ginseng. Asian ginseng is an adaptogen and has been valued for centuries for its ability to improve both physical and mental abilities, such as memory, concentration, thinking, physical stamina, and endurance. These benefits have made panax ginseng a popular herb for helping people cope with stress, depression, and anxiety, and it is even used to relieve sleeping problems, pain, headache, and stomach disorders.

Just because Asian ginseng has been used for centuries for the conditions I've already mentioned does not mean scientists have verified the claims.

Fortunately, some studies have been done, and thus far there is some evidence that Asian ginseng has an ability to reduce stress as well as thinking and reaction times. For example, thirty healthy volunteers were randomly assigned to take either placebo or Asian ginseng (200 mg or 400 mg daily) for eight days, followed by a six-day "holiday" period. This was a crossover study, which means all the subjects participated in each of the three dosing possibilities. The researchers discovered that taking 200 mg of Asian ginseng helped with mood while the 400 mg dose improved calmness.

One challenge with Asian ginseng is quality: this herb is costly so be sure to get the supplement from a reputable manufacturer. You should also check with an independent quality control organization, such as Consumer Labs, for reports on the quality of Asian ginseng, as well as other supplements. Once you find a reputable brand, the suggested dose is typically 200 mg daily of an extract standardized to contain 4 percent to 7 percent ginsenosides, which are the active ingredients in this herb.

Although Asian ginseng is considered to be a safe herb, experts recommend taking it for two to three weeks and then taking a one to two-week "holiday" before starting it again, if needed. Asian ginseng may interact with insulin or oral antidiabetes drugs (you may need to change your drug dose; ask your doctor) and the herb may also reduce the effects of warfarin (Coumadin).

Ashwagandha
One of the most popular herbs in Ayurvedic medicine is ashwagandha (*Withania somnifera*), which has been valued for thousands of years for its restorative abilities. Among its features are the ability to help the body fight off the negative impact of stress, improve mood, and boost the immune system. Ashwagandha, which belongs to the same family as the tomato, contains a variety of medicinal components, including withanolides, alkaloids, choline,

amino acids, and fatty acids. The ashwagandha root is the part of the plant most often used in herbal remedies, although the leaves and fruit also have healing qualities.

The typical dose of ashwagandha is 600 to 1,000 mg taken twice a day. To help with stress, anxiety, and insomnia, you can mix one teaspoon of powdered ashwagandha into a cup of hot nonfat milk or soymilk before bedtime. Ashwagandha is a safe herb, but at extremely high doses it has been reported to cause miscarriages in animals. Therefore, as a precaution, pregnant women should not take ashwagandha, although no similar studies have been done in humans. Talk to your health-care provider before taking ashwagandha, especially if you have a medical condition such as diabetes (ashwagandha may help lower glucose levels), heart disease, thyroid disease, or autoimmune disorders such as lupus or rheumatoid arthritis.

Schizandra berry

What do you call a remedy that tastes acrid, bitter, salty, sour, and sweet, all at the same time? The answer is schizandra (or schisandra; *Schisandra chinensis, S. arisanensis, S. rubriflora*), also referred to as the "five-flavored seed" by the Chinese. Schizandra berries have been part of the Chinese medicine world for thousands of years and highly valued for their ability to relieve stress and anxiety, boost energy, support the immune system, improve mental clarity, and help liver function. According to Donald R. Yance, Jr., author of *Herbal Medicine, Healing and Cancer,* schizandra has the ability to stimulate your central nervous system and boost your mental abilities in a positive, calm manner, without causing the jitters.

What does the science say? So far the studies of schizandra and stress have been done in mice, but according to the results, the herb is effective at relieving stress levels. A study published in *Phytomedicine* in October 2011 reported on the effect of schizandra extract in stressed mice, noting that the herb "reversed stress-induced anxiety level" and also caused changes in brain chemicals associated with stress. An earlier study, also in mice, found that a combination of schizandra and Baikel skullcap (a calming herb) "could be used to treat stress disorders," according to the researchers.

If you are interested in trying schizandra extract, look for a standardized extract containing 3.4 percent schisandrin (an active ingredient in the fruit). A typical dose range for managing stress is 1.5 to 6 grams daily, so it's best to start low and increase the dose gradually to see how you respond. Side effects are uncommon and may include upset stomach, heartburn, itching, and rash.

Other Stress-Reducing Herbs

Other herbs that may help calm the body and mind include chamomile (*Matricaria chamomilla*), kava kava (*Piper methysticum*), and valerian (*Valeriana officinalis*). When making herbal tea with fresh or dried herbs, boil the water, turn it off, and then let the herbs steep in the hot water for five to fifteen minutes.

Chamomile, also known as German chamomile, is an annual plant in the same family as ragweed and daisies. This popular herb has been used for millennia to treat insomnia, anxiety, stomach cramps, and rashes, among other ailments. The flowers of chamomile are used to make the remedies, and the most popular form of the herb is chamomile tea. The calming effect of chamomile is credited to a flavonoid in the plant called aplgenin, which has an ability to attach to certain sedative receptors in the brain.

When brewing chamomile tea from fresh or dried flowers, use two to three teaspoons of the herb for each eight ounces of water. If you purchase chamomile tea in tea bags, some brands offer a mixture of chamomile and other herbs or flavors, such as peppermint or cinnamon. If you are allergic to ragweed, daisies, or mums, you may have an allergic reaction to chamomile tea. Although side effects associated with chamomile are rare, the herb may increase the risk of bleeding, so do not use it if you are taking blood-thinning medications or supplements. Do not use chamomile if you are pregnant or while drinking alcohol.

Kava kava is typically used to treat anxiety and to help with insomnia and other sleep problems. The active ingredient in kava kava is called kavalactone, and any kava kava supplement you take should contain a standardized extract of 30 percent kavalactone. A common dose of kava kava to relieve stress is 250 mg (by capsule or one-half dropperful of liquid) three times daily with meals. For help with sleep, a typical dose is up to 1,500 mg, but you should not take kava kava for more than four months continuously because of the rare possibility of liver problems. Do not use kava kava if you are pregnant and do not use it with alcohol.

Valerian is another herb frequently used to help with insomnia, anxiety, and stress. The valerian plant is a flowering perennial whose roots are used for herbal remedies. You can mix one teaspoon of powdered valerian root in sixteen ounces of boiling water and let it steep for ten minutes before using. The taste of valerian root tea may take a while to get used to, but if you add a little honey, the taste improves.

To help with sleep, valerian should be taken about thirty to forty-five minutes before bedtime, typically 150 mg (standardized extract of 0.8 percent valeric acid, an active ingredient in valerian). If this dose is not helpful, you can gradually increase it to 600 mg per night, but talk to your doctor before using this herb. Valerian root should not be used for more than four weeks continuously, and you should gradually decrease your dose before stopping completely. Possible side effects may include stomachache, headache, and drowsiness after waking up. Do not take valerian root if you are pregnant or when using alcohol.

STRESS-BUSTING TEA RECIPES

Here are two stress-busting herbal tea recipes that may help before bedtime or anytime you need to "chill out."

   1/3 teaspoon rosemary leaves
   1/4 teaspoon dried sage
   1/4 teaspoon skullcap powder
   1/6 teaspoon powdered valerian root

Steep the mixture of these herbs in 8 ounces of boiling water and drink before bedtime.

Another stress-busting tea is even easier to make:

   1/2 teaspoon dried lemon balm
   1/2 teaspoon dried peppermint

HOMEOPATHIC REMEDIES FOR STRESS

Another natural approach to managing the stress in your life is the use of homeopathic remedies. Many people are skeptical of homeopathic remedies, and one reason is that there are limited scientific studies to support their use. However, that attitude may be changing slowly as more research is being conducted into the use of combination homeopathic remedies. This combination approach is a shift from classical homeopathy, in which a homeopath determines which single remedy will work best for an individual based on that person's characteristics and profile.

In addition, however, high-quality homeopathic remedies are now available that have been formulated to contain ingredients specifically for a given ailment or set of similar symptoms. For example, if you are experiencing stress, anxiety, and insomnia, one homeopathic product on the market contains *Matricaria chamomilla* (chamomile), *Humulus lupulus* (hops), *Passiflora incarnata* (passionflower), *Valeriana officinalis* (valerian root), *Coffea cruda* (unroasted coffee beans), and several other ingredients. These are natural substances that can be found in the *Homeopathic Pharmacopoeia of the United States*, the master publication that contains monographs and other information about the various substances used in homeopathic remedies, as well as the standards for manufacturing homeopathic remedies.

Homeopathic remedies dissolve easily under the tongue and can be used safely with other nutritional supplements. If you choose to take homeopathic remedies, follow the directions on the label or consult a knowledgeable naturopath or homeopath.

Another option is to consult a classical homeopath, who will conduct a thorough interview with you to help identify the most appropriate homeopathic remedy for your needs.

AROMATHERAPY AND ESSENTIAL OILS FOR STRESS

Smell is the only one of your senses that can break through the blood barrier to the central nervous system. That's why the smell of apple pie may evoke memories of baking with your grandmother, or the fragrance of a certain cologne can bring back memories of a specific person or event.

Thus aromatherapy and the use of essential oils shown to produce a calming effect can be an effective tool in managing and reducing stress and anxiety, and also help with sleep. Essential oils are concentrated liquids that are extracted from plants. Also known as volatile oils and ethereal oils, they contain volatile aroma compounds and are called essential because they have a specific essence of the plant from which they are derived.

How Essential Oils Work

Essential oils in aromatherapy can be used in three different ways: inhalation, topical application, and orally. I will discuss the first two only. When the oils are applied to the skin, you get benefits from inhaling them, so let's start with inhalation. Experts are still uncertain exactly how aromatherapy works, but they have some theories.

One idea is that as fragrances enter the nose, the smell receptors transmit signals to areas of the brain, specifically the amygdala and hippocampus, which are where memories and emotions are processed and stored. The molecules of essential oils may stimulate these brain areas and have an impact on emotional and physical well-being, similar to how medications used to treat anxiety and stress work. Others believe essential oil molecules may have an impact on enzymes or hormones in the body.

The activity of essential oils is different when they are applied to the skin. Essential oils are fat soluble and have a small molecular structure, which make it easy for them to pass through the skin and into the surrounding tissues and bloodstream. Before applying nearly all essential oils, it is critical that you dilute them with a carrier oil, such as olive, jojoba, or almond oil, or other vegetable or nut oil. Undiluted essential oils can cause skin irritations, such as burning, itching, or rashes. The typical dilution formula is 40 drops of essential oil per 1 ounce of carrier oil, which translates into 5 percent essential oil and 95 percent carrier oil. Two essential oils that can be applied to the skin without dilution are lavender and chamomile, while two that should not be used topically at all (unless under a professional's supervision) are cinnamon oil and oregano oil. All others should be diluted as noted.

A limited number of scientific studies have been done on the effectiveness of essential oils in managing stress or anxiety. For example, a pilot study was done involving twenty-eight postpartum women at a large Indianapolis hospital. Half the women were treated with inhalation aromatherapy consisting of lavender and rose essential oils twice a week for fifteen minutes per session for four weeks while the other half were asked to avoid all aromatherapy for four weeks. At the end of the four weeks, the women who were treated with aromatherapy had significantly better scores on tests for generalized anxiety and depression than did the women who were not treated.

Another study involved the use of two of the more popular essential oils used for stress and anxiety—lavender and bergamot. The combination of these oils or a placebo was applied to the abdomen of forty healthy volunteers, each of whom had their blood pressure, breathing rate, pulse rate, and skin temperature checked before and after application of the oils. All the volunteers also were questioned about their emotional state.

Compared with those who received the placebo, the volunteers who were treated with essential oils had a significantly lower blood pressure and pulse rate. People in the essential oil group also reported being "more calm" and "more relaxed" than people in the control group. The authors of the study determined that "this synergistic blend provides evidence for its use in medicine for treating depression or anxiety in humans."

How to Enjoy Essential Oils

In addition to lavender and bergamot oils, several other essential oils may be helpful. Aromatherapists generally recommend the following choices for dealing with stress and sleep issues:

For stress and anxiety. Most effective are bergamot, chamomile, lemon, marjoram, and sandalwood. Others that may be helpful include basil, cypress, frankincense, geranium, jonquil, juniper, neroli.

For sleep problems. Chamomile, lemon, marjoram, neroli, rose, valerian.

You can use essential oils in a variety of ways. Consider one or more of these options, and remember to dilute any oils you use topically as noted above.

- Use diluted essential oils as part of an acupressure or massage session.

- Rub lavender oil or chamomile oil into the bottom tip of the sternum, which is known as the solar plexus, to relieve tension.

- Make your stress-reducing aromatherapy portable by placing a few small pieces of rock salt into a vial or small bottle and then adding a few drops of your favorite essential oil. The rock salt will absorb the oil and provide you with a convenient pick-me-up wherever you go!

- Place 4 to 5 drops of essential oil into 8 ounces of water in a spritzer bottle and use it in your home or workplace.

- Add 5 to 10 drops of essential oil to a warm bath and relax!

- Add several drops of essential oil to a diffuser. There are several types of essential oil diffusers, including electric and nonelectric models. All are designed to dispense a continuous stream of fragrance over a wide area. They are convenient and often attractive and can be placed in any room in the house or office.

Do not use essential oil if you are pregnant or have asthma. Consult your health-care provider about aromatherapy if you have allergies.

STEP 5

Express Yourself

Okay, now it's time for the fun chapter, the one where you reach down deep inside yourself and express who you are in creative, exciting, fun, and stress-banishing ways.

Did I hear you say you're not creative, or that you're not artistic? Or, as one woman named Clara said to me, "I don't have an artistic bone in my body." More than likely that's not true; you probably just have not allowed your creative energy to be released or realized. This turned out to be the case for Clara. With a little prodding, it turned out Clara had a deep-seated desire to do flower arranging and experiment with bonsai, yet she felt as if she were "stuck" in a large bank, where she processed mortgage applications, so she shut down and suppressed her inner desires.

You can redirect the energy you now dedicate to fighting the stressors and anxiety in your life and channel it in ways that enlighten, develop, and enhance your body, mind, and spirit. When women refocus their energies by embracing their creative spirit, they can transform the anxiety, uncertainty, and stress in their lives into something positive, a mode of self-healing, empowerment, and discovery.

So, how do you express yourself? Or two better questions might be, "How do you *want* to express yourself?" and "When are you going to start?" In this chapter, you will learn about the relationship between creativity and stress and how to identify and harness your creative energies so you can banish your anxieties and discover the self-healing powers of your inner spirit.

CREATIVITY AND STRESS

In a study published in the *Journal of Aging and Health* in June 2012, the lead researcher, Nicholas Turiano, explained several important benefits associated with creativity. Results of the study, which involved more than one thousand older men, indicated that creative people have a superior ability to handle stress. Turiano noted that "creative people may see stressors more as challenges that they can work to overcome rather than as stressful obstacles they can't overcome." This may explain why individuals with a creative streak tend to remain calmer in emotionally or physically stressful situations, he said. Therefore, people who engage in creative activities may reduce stress and stimulate their brain, thereby improving or enhancing their health.

Another advantage associated with creativity is a reduced risk of dying. In fact, creativity was a greater indicator of a longer life span than were overall openness and intelligence in this study. According to Turiano, one possible reason for this finding is that creativity enhances health because it engages many different neural networks in the brain. He pointed out that "individuals high in creativity maintain the integrity of their neural networks even into old age." This concept and similar ones have been supported by other research.

In fact, a British researcher conducted a systematic review of eleven studies of creative activities and their impact on mental health and made the following statement: "The evidence suggests that creative activities can have a healing and protective effect on mental well-being. Their therapeutic effects promote relaxation, provide a means of self-expression, reduce blood pressure while boosting the immune system and reducing stress."

Rachel's Story

Rachel was fifty-six years old when I met her in 2012, and she had been working as a veterinary assistant since 1998. She said her job was both emotionally stressful and fulfilling, and her love of animals extended to her off-work hours as well, as she lived with four dogs and three cats. Her second marriage had ended in divorce five years earlier, and she was currently dating, but it was "nothing serious."

When our discussion turned to stress and creativity, she quickly dismissed the idea. "I don't have time, and besides, I really don't know what I'd do. My work and my animals are my life." She admitted liking jazz and was an avid reader, and said her best form of stress relief was jogging nearly every day, which she did with two of her dogs.

"But you know something," she said just before I was about to leave, "I remember on nine-eleven, I felt really helpless and anxious, and I did something strange." Rachel said she retrieved a box of unusual shells she had collected years earlier on her honeymoon and spent the next two days creating a wall hanging on canvas. She pointed to the final product, which was on her living room wall.

"Somehow, making that wall hanging made me feel more at peace," she said. "Sometimes I look at it and wonder if I'd ever do something like that again." I suggested she had found a road to her creative spirit, and that perhaps she could combine her love of animals with that creative process.

It had taken more than a decade, but Rachel finally realized she was harboring a kernel of creative energy that would allow her to manage her stress and feel good about herself. She has been following that energy and is now creating mixed-media wall hangings with animals as her theme.

THE HEALING POWER OF CREATIVE THERAPY

While art therapy usually refers to activities such as drawing and painting, a broader, more encompassing term now used in some circles is creative therapy. The concept of creative therapy includes activities such as playing the flute or drums, molding clay, writing poetry, or tap dancing as a way to relieve stress and nurture one's creativity.

The healing power of creativity stems from its ability to help people become so engrossed in the activity they have chosen, they completely put aside their stress and anxiety for a while. During the time you are dedicated to and concentrating on the creative process, your body, mind, and spirit release the tension they have been harboring. You can become one with the activity, whether it's dancing, writing, painting, sculpting, or carving.

"When I'm writing poetry," says Cleo, a thirty-three-year-old part-time bartender and part-time dog groomer, "I'm somewhere else. I forget time. I feel like I become one with the words and their meaning. Writing poetry is meditative and exciting and even frustrating at times, but a good frustration, because I get energized by the power of the poem. Writing poetry also allows me to take any anger, hopelessness, or other negative feelings I have and channel them into something beautiful. I guess that's the healing power of poetry for me."

In a way, engaging in the creative process is like meditation, because it allows you to focus your attention on something specific and positive for an extended period of time. Creative activities can help you feel good about yourself and your place in your family, at your workplace, and in the world.

FINDING AND RELEASING YOUR CREATIVE SPIRIT

One underlying frustration and stress-producing factor in women's live is unrealized, suppressed creativity. Do you ever watch young children coloring with crayons and wish you could color too? Let's hope you joined in! Allow yourself to tap in to your creative side and discover the stress-reducing and spirit-lifting power of that energy.

Do you know what your creative energy is? There are scores of possibilities, and only you will know the right fit. There's no right or wrong answer. If your creative activity enhances your mental, physical, emotional, and spiritual well-being, then it's the correct choice for you.

Have you suppressed your creative juices? Do you secretly want to learn ballet, paint watercolor landscapes, sing with a rock band, or create papier-mâché masks? If the stress of always doing the "right thing" and working hard to conform to other people's expectations has quashed your dreams, it's time to take back control, organize your time, prioritize, and devote time to nurturing your spirit and your emotions. It's time to release the tension that has built up inside of you, to express yourself and play. Once you give yourself permission to take this step, you will enjoy a sense of fulfillment, release stress, and become a more satisfied, balanced, and productive person.

Getting Started

Do you feel like you need a boost to get your creative juices flowing? Are you unsure about where your creative energies lie? If you have repressed your creative side or been afraid or just too busy with work and family and other obligations to explore this other side of yourself, then you need some icebreakers. The popular theory has been that the right side of the brain is the home of creativity and intuition, although there are some experts who now say the left side plays a critical role in these processes as well—so don't discount any part of the brain when it comes to being creative.

If you need some help identifying or finding your creative kernel of energy, here are a few tips:

- Meditate or use breathing exercises. Both of these methods will help you relax and release tension. It's difficult to get into a creative frame of mind if you are tense and your mind is racing. Tips on meditation and breathing exercises are in step 3.

- Write it down. You may want to have a pen and paper handy when meditating or doing breathing exercises so you can jot down your thoughts. Even if you don't use these relaxation approaches, writing down your thoughts is an excellent way to help make your dreams real and also allow you to examine all the possibilities and see where they lead you.

- Picture yourself being creative. Sit someplace quiet and allow your mind to imagine you are doing the creative activities you have thought about or written down. Consider all the angles of each project, including what you need to achieve it and where you can do it. This is a good time to use visualization, drawing upon sights, sounds, smells, and touch to make each experience as real as possible. During this process, you may realize whether this creative project is something that will satisfy you or whether you have some misgivings or worries associated with it. It can be helpful to jot down your feelings during these sessions so you can remember how you felt about each idea.

- Allow yourself to feel. Don't worry about what other people may think about the type of creative road you want to take. This process is about you and how you can expand your spirit and better manage the stress in your life. If you want to write short stories, paint pictures of flowers, or learn how to make cheese, go for it. Do you remember how you felt as a child when you created something—a picture you may have drawn for your parents, clay figures you made in class, leaves and flowers you dried between the pages of books, and little stories you wrote and illustrated with crayons? Remember the joy of those occasions? You can get in touch with those feelings again. What's important is that you take the first step and identify your creative passion and then get ready to pursue it.

Pursuing Your Creative Choice

Hopefully the previous tips have helped you prepare to launch into the next step, which is the actual pursuit of your creative streak. If you have identified more than one activity you wish to pursue, select the one you feel most comfortable with or the one that inspires you the most. Then go for it!

Depending on what type of project you have chosen, you may want to take a class, attend a lecture (either real or online), talk to professionals in the field, read books or watch videos on the topic, or explore the topic further in other ways. Immerse yourself in the idea, and then you'll discover whether it will work for you.

Here are some general guidelines on how to pursue your creative choice:

- Do it every day. Dedicate a block of time every day, thirty to sixty minutes if possible, to pursue your activity. If you have decided to learn French, for example, listen to tapes or online classes, read a beginning French language book, or practice repeating phrases. If you have started a journal, be sure to write in it every day, even if you don't think you have anything to say—write about that!

- Diversify. Consider pursuing your creative adventure via a variety of avenues. For example, if you have decided to write short stories, see if there is a writing group in your area you can join, attend a lecture or classes on short story writing (real or virtual online classes or talks), or set as a goal to submit one of your stories to a contest. Have you taken up photography? Attend photography showings, find a photography club in your city, or make it a habit to study the styles of different photographers past and present.

- Don't judge yourself. You don't need to be an accomplished painter, musician, photographer, dancer, baker, or linguist. Just release and enjoy your creative energy without labeling it good or bad, right or wrong. Your creations can be just for you or for others—it's up to you. If you are not comfortable showing or telling others what you are doing, then don't do so until you are ready. The important thing is that you are nurturing an essential part of yourself and releasing "stuff" that you need to give up so you can feel better physical, emotionally, mentally, and spiritually.

- Give yourself time. Practice and engage in your creative activity for at least three to six weeks before you make any decisions about whether it feels right for you and whether you wish to continue pursuing it. Be honest—but not hard!—with yourself. If you took up playing the guitar and are struggling with reading music but realize it's going to take more time before you improve, then good for you, so keep going! If, however, you have tried painting flowers and feel increasingly frustrated and stressed over what you perceive to be failures, then it's time to reevaluate your choice of creativity. It's possible you may feel more confident painting something else or trying another artistic medium, such as working with clay, making collages, or creating papier-mâché animals or masks and painting them.

- Branch out. Feel free to try more than one creative adventure or try something that may complement the choice you have made already. You may find that once you let your creativity out of the closet, you will want to pursue even more opportunities.

- Stay out of touch. That's right; turn off the cell phone and the landline while you are engaged in your creative process. I promise you won't be naked without the phone strapped to your belt.

- Keep a journal. If your creative process involves a journal, then this tip is redundant, but if not, then it can be helpful to keep a written record of your feelings and ideas about your creative process in a journal. Maintaining a journal is an excellent way to keep track of creative ideas, sketches, dreams, and your feelings.

- Create and maintain a blog. This tip isn't for everyone, but some people are energized by keeping a blog and sharing their ideas and feelings with a wider community. Keeping a blog also can be viewed as a commitment, which may be a positive or negative element, depending on how you perceive it. Some people find that keeping a blog is good discipline and forces them (in a positive way) to keep writing, creating, and sharing, which ultimately helps with their stress. Others, however, may feel more stress associated with keeping a blog, in which case this may not be a good choice.

- Explore online opportunities. Regardless of which creative activity you have chosen, there are likely thousands of Web sites related to it in some way. There are sites that offer free guitar lessons, tips on how to grow bonsai, information on poetry and short story contests to enter, videos on how to tap-dance, instructions on how to make a quilt, and online forums where you can chat with others who are also pursuing your activity; it's all out there, waiting for you. One beauty of the Internet is twenty-four hour access. When you have long stretches of time to explore, great! But if you can't sleep, if you have a few free moments before you leave for work in the morning, if you're waiting for your kids to get ready for school, you might go online and check out a new artist, practice speaking French, or watch a short video on piano-playing techniques.

- Meditate on your choices. After you have spent several months nurturing your creative spirit, occasionally take some time to meditate on what the experiences mean to you and how they have changed your perspective on life and your stress level.

I have mentioned meditation at least twice in this section, and now here I'm bringing it up again. However, this variant of meditation is more passive. It's the meditative state that people often enter into when they are engaged in creative activities. Many people, and not just professional artists and the like, find they become completely engrossed during the creative process, whether they are dancing, drawing, writing, sculpting, carving, or building something.

"I lose all track of time when I'm creating collages," says Tabitha. "It's like each piece of fabric, shell, bead, piece of paper—each item takes on a life of its own and I become one with the process of creating the collage. My collages are personal statements about life, and I feel like I'm communicating with the piece as I'm creating it, and so I seem to enter another world, just me and the collage."

This type of meditative escape is just what the doctor ordered to help shed stress in your life. It's like a minivacation that you can take without the need for tickets or getting in the car.

Here's a final tip on channeling your creative energy: do it at work. If you experience stress on the job, let your creative spirit come out to play during a coffee break or during lunch. Write a poem, do some sketches, read an article about bonsai, listen to language tapes, take a walk and look for collage materials, or watch a short video on the Internet about your artistic pursuit. Tapping into your creativity while on the job can help lift some of the tension from your day.

CREATIVE STRESS RELIEF

Do you need some help getting your creative juices flowing? Here are a few ideas you can try. You'll need safety goggles for one of them!

- Get a large piece of paper and something to draw with—pencils, pens, crayons, or markers. Sit at a desk or other large flat surface where you can spread out the paper—butcher paper is great because you can cover a large surface with it. Find a place where you can be undisturbed and alone for about fifteen to twenty minutes and sit quietly. Close your eyes, breathe gently and deeply, and focus on the stressful situation in your life. Begin to draw what the situation feels like or looks like to you—but keep your eyes closed. Just let your drawing instrument flow over the paper as you release your feelings onto the paper. Don't worry about what your drawing looks like: it's meant to portray your emotions, not be a piece of art. When you feel like you're done, open your eyes. Meditate for a few minutes on what you have drawn and how you feel about it.

- You might need safety goggles for this exercise. An artist I met told me that she uses this technique occasionally and that she always feels better after she is done. She collects old damaged ceramic plates, mugs, and other similar items, and when she is stressed, she spreads them out

continued

on a large sheet in her garage, covers them with another sheet, dons her goggles, and then smashes the ceramics with a hammer. Since she creates mosaics, she uses some of the pieces for her artwork, and leftovers she uses in her garden. Another artist confessed to smashing ceramic coffee mugs against the brick wall in the back of her yard and then crushing the bigger pieces with a hammer. While a bit extreme, both women claimed this was a great stress reducer—and productive too!

• You may have heard the expression "hopping mad." Why not hop and dance away your stress? Hide in a room (with a lock if necessary), turn up the music (or wear earphones), and let go. You can dance and sing, pretend you're a rock or country star, and let out all your feelings. The woman who shared this idea with me says she sometimes does this several times a week for about ten minutes each time, and it makes her feel great. It's also wonderful exercise.

WHAT THE EXPERTS SAY

Some researchers have compared different creative processes to determine their physiological impact. One such study was done with thirty female and twenty-seven male college students who participated in one of four different thirty-minute sessions: playing the piano, molding clay, writing calligraphy, and remaining silent. The study's authors found that cortisol levels, which were measured both before and after the sessions, were markedly lower in the three creative activity groups when compared with the silent group, while playing the piano showed the most significant decline in the stress hormone.

Art Therapy

The power of art therapy to help people ranging from very young children to the elderly deal with stress, trauma, and depression is well documented. Art therapy is recognized as a legitimate tool to help individuals resolve personal and interpersonal conflicts and problems, reduce stress, modify their behavior, raise self-awareness and self-esteem, and realize their full potential on every level. You don't need to see an art therapist or other mental health professional to enjoy the therapeutic benefits of art, but that is another option you can pursue (see step 7). Art therapy is a tool some therapists use to help their clients cope with the stress in their lives.

In the United Kingdom, in fact, people who experience stress, depression, or anxiety and who visit their doctor may walk out of the office with a prescription, not for an antidepressant or other mood-modifying drug, but for art therapy through a program called Arts on Prescription. Experts point out that the program, which is available throughout the country, helps people "through creativity and increasing social engagement," and that the "creative activities take place in the community facilitated by artists rather than therapists."

Dance!

Although dance involves physical activity, it also is a form of creative expression and a great way to reduce stress, and so I have included it in this chapter. Although other forms of physical exercise may be said to involve some amount of personal expression and emotion, none can make that claim quite like dance can. Dance has been used as part of religious, ceremonial, and social events for millennia, and in many cultures, including Native American, dance has been an integral part of healing ceremonies.

Today, dance therapy is recognized as a valid complementary therapy for individuals who are recovering from chronic physical, emotional, and mental illness and disease. Dance helps heal on two levels: physically by improving flexibility, mobility, coordination, and balance; and emotionally/mentally by releasing tension and anxiety, improving self-esteem and self-awareness, and allowing a creative outlet for emotions.

One of my favorite studies on the effects of dance on stress included the tango. The study included nearly sixty-six women and men ages eighteen to eighty who said they were experiencing stress, depression, and anxiety. All the participants were randomly assigned to one of three groups: tango, mindfulness meditation (see step 3), or control group. Individuals in the dance and meditation groups attended ninety-minute sessions once a week for six weeks.

Stress, anxiety, and depression levels were measured both before and after the test period. People who participated in the tango classes or meditation classes showed a significant reduction in depression when compared with controls, but only those in the tango group also had a significant reduction in stress. The study's lead author, Rosa Pinniger, a psychologist at the University of New England in Australia, noted that "even tango music is proposed to generate positive emotions."

Can't dance? Think you have two left feet? If you'd like to try dancing but are afraid you'll make a fool of yourself, you're not alone. However, you can prepare for dance lessons by borrowing a DVD or tape from the library or watching YouTube or other videos online and become familiar with the basics before you attempt lessons.

Broaden your horizons when it comes to dance. Ballroom dancing can be great fun, but don't overlook ballet, salsa, hip-hop, belly dancing, square dancing, clogging, and zumba.

STEP 6

Socialize

Women tend to have a natural ability to bring people and other living things together. Overall, women do most of the child rearing, are more likely to care for aging parents, are typically the driving force in arranging family gatherings and reunions, and tend to be matchmakers—both professionally and as a matter of fact. I'm not saying these things to be sexist—it's just the way it seems to be. Women can capitalize on this bonding and socializing strength and ability to help them reduce and manage the stress in their lives.

In a July 2012 article in *Psychology Today* on stress,

Teri L. Bourdeau, professor at the Oklahoma State University Center for Health Sciences, explained that "there are more people working later in life and thus are more engaged in activities that require cognitive engagement and socializing. It is well-known that good social supports aid in management of stress."

You can use the power of socializing to rein in your stress levels. In this chapter, I have broadened the use of the term "socialize" to include how women interact with friends and family, the natural world, and the community at large, which includes the Internet. Here you can explore how you can use these venues to deal with the stressors in your life.

HOW SOCIALIZING REDUCES STRESS

The adages about "no man is an island" and about how humans are social creatures are true. Aside from rare exceptions, people tend to seek the company of and connect with other people to varying degrees. (I often think of the movie *Castaway* with Tom Hanks and how, faced with living alone on the island, he painted a face on a basketball and named him Wilson.) This natural desire to make and maintain human connections plays an important role in reducing stress, anxiety, and fear in our lives. There is safety, security, and comfort in joining the company of other people, even if it is virtual, as we can do so easily today via the Internet. Chat rooms and forums allow everyone with computer access an opportunity to reach out and be part of a larger community.

These new developments in socializing don't mean the "old-fashioned way" of calling people on the phone, writing letters, or meeting in person aren't still important— they are, and perhaps more than ever, since many people miss these more personal ways of connecting. But technology has provided us with additional ways to stay in touch with others and to feel less lonely, isolated, and insecure.

One remarkable woman I met and spoke with about stress and socializing is Priscilla, an eighty-four-year-old retired social worker who lives alone, still drives and does her own shopping, and who, in her own words, is "having so much fun" taking classes, attending lectures, and meeting and talking with new people all the time. Every day is an adventure, she says, and she wishes she had more hours in the day to do all the things she wants to do.

Priscilla does all of her socializing from her home, sitting in front of one of her two computers. She watches and listens to lectures from major universities, participates in a number of different chat rooms and forums on topics such as politics, religion, and education, and corresponds with a range of people around the world on these and other topics. Whenever she feels stressed or anxious about events in the world, financial matters, or other concerns, she searches for answers to her questions on the Internet, poses questions to people she has met online, and seeks out other resources to solve her problems.

"I live alone and rarely have visitors, and that is my choice, yet I'm never lonely," she says. "My life is full of people and ideas, and I'm always learning something new. My advice to people, especially older people who may be homebound or who can't get out as much as they used to, and who feel stressed or isolated, is to connect with other people on the Internet. There's a whole world out there, and you can bring it into your home with a computer."

Priscilla has found an excellent way to socialize while remaining safe and secure in her own home. Seeking out and maintaining social contacts while using a computer is one way to socialize, and a convenient one for many people for a variety of reasons. But at least for now, there's one thing socializing via cyberspace does not allow you to do, and that is physically touch the other person or persons in your social circle. As you'll see here, something special happens at a hormonal and molecular level when people touch each other.

Socializing and Hormones

Socialization is a critical factor in physical, emotional, and spiritual health. On a physical level, for example, maintaining social contact seems to have an impact on hormone balance. One hormone involved in socialization and stress is oxytocin. Studies indicate that maintaining an adequate level of socializing results in higher levels of oxytocin, which in turn works to lower anxiety and stimulate the parasympathetic nervous system's ability to induce a sense of calm.

In fact, oxytocin is often referred to as the "love" or "trust" hormone because higher levels are associated with an increased desire to socialize and to form relationships and connections with other people. People who are experiencing stress in their lives but who also maintain a regular level of social contact and support get an oxytocin boost, which in turns helps them feel more confident, less anxious, and more willing to socialize. Therefore, there is a positive cycle associated with social support, oxytocin, and stress.

Scientists have witnessed how mice exposed to stress in a social situation (forced to live in crowded living quarters) showed much less stress and anxiety when given oxytocin. But people don't have to be given oxytocin: they can get it by simply reaching out and hugging someone or offering to hold their hand. If you spoon with your partner in bed, both you and your partner's brain release a small amount of oxytocin. When you take the hand of your child, parent, or grandchild, you both release oxytocin. If you don't have a human to hug, that's all right too. Oxytocin is also released when you hug your cat or dog. Thus the mere act of making bodily contact establishes trust, love, and comfort—all great antidotes for stress and anxiety.

Pumping out some oxytocin also can help reduce levels of the stress hormone cortisol and help lower blood pressure. Oxytocin and receptors for the hormone have even been found in the intestinal tract, which could explain why it also provides relief from gastrointestinal discomfort.

Socializing and Caring

When you socialize with other people, you tend to focus on others rather than yourself. Even if your reason for getting together with other people is to have someone who will listen to your problems or to commiserate with you, some of the focus will be directed outward. In return for sharing with others, you may get some understanding, sympathy, emotional assistance, and love. Your problems and worries may become less burdensome and you may feel wanted, cared for, and part of a larger social network. Feelings of despair or hopelessness that may accompany stress and anxiety can be alleviated when you share your concerns with others and hear their perspectives as well. Of course, much of the good emotions associated with socializing may be happening without you consciously realizing it at the time.

"It's happened to me on numerous occasions," says Rebecca, a forty-eight-year-old library clerk. "I'm feeling on edge and stressed, yet I have an event to attend, a family gathering, or something to do for the library, and I really don't want to go. I feel like I don't have the time to be away from what I think I need to do. But when I do go, I nearly always leave feeling better. Even if I never mention anything that's bothering me or the difficulties in my life, I leave the gathering feeling more uplifted and, frankly, better able to cope with my problems. Being with people is like a shot in the arm or an affirmation for me."

Like any journey, the first step toward socializing or inviting others into your home or circle can be the most difficult one. You're stressed, you're miserable, you have too much to do, and you want to be left alone. Sometimes these can be valid reasons for avoiding social situations, but it's also critical to reach out and get that oxytocin flowing! So here are a few suggestions on how you can increase your socialization skills:

- Introduce yourself to others. If you go to an event such as a lecture or art show and you don't know anyone, do you tend to be a wallflower or slip out of the event as soon as it's over to avoid speaking with people? Or do you introduce yourself to someone you may recognize but not by name, or walk up to a complete stranger and introduce yourself and make a comment about the program or show? Naturally, you should use discretion when talking to strangers, but there are typically many opportunities to socialize at events even when you don't know anyone. Thank the host or hostess, ask a question about the event or the food, or seek more information about future programs.

- Initiate social gatherings. Such events don't have to be elaborate or time-consuming, but they can be healthful social opportunities that might help relieve some of the stress in your life. Be the one to suggest getting together for coffee, a walk, a picnic lunch, an informal dinner, or a few hours at the beach or around the pool.

• Join a group of like-minded people. Do you have a hobby or an interest in art, swimming, religion or spirituality, music, or other topics? Getting together with others who share your interests is a great way to socialize and perhaps also expand your knowledge or experience in certain areas. (Step 5, "Express Yourself," explores this aspect of stress management from a creative perspective in detail.)

• Stay in touch. How often do you communicate with your best friends, relatives, and other special people in your life? Taking a few moments on a regular basis to call a friend just to say hello and check in with them, or even sending an e-mail or text message (although less personal) are other ways to socialize and feel part of the larger circle.

• Learn to say no. Although it's important to socialize as a way to reduce stress, it's equally important to recognize when to say no to social events. These are times when you need to be completely honest with yourself: are you going to say no to a social gathering because you truly believe attending will raise your stress level or because the individual has been making unreasonable demands on your time? If the answer is yes, then declining is probably appropriate. If people begin to place uncomfortable demands on your relationship, then it's time to set the *P* in DROP into motion—prioritize—and learn how to say no (see chapter 1). If you don't, you will likely find yourself experiencing even more stress in your relationship with this individual.

- Remember that quality is better than quantity. When it comes to effectively reducing stress and feeling confident about a relationship with someone, it's more important to stay in touch with a few close friends than it is to surround yourself with lots of acquaintances or people you don't know very well. The quality of a relationship also depends on the amount of give-and-take (reciprocity) between you and the other person. Maintaining a healthy balance between listening to and supporting another individual and having that person also listen and support you takes effort on the part of both parties. But as you've likely experienced if you have a best friend, that effort reaps big rewards.

- Don't discount virtual socialization. The Internet offers a wealth of opportunities to socialize virtually: in chat rooms and forums, through lectures and classes, and via e-mail and Skype. You can make friends around the world and share stories, photos, and real-time face-to-face communication if you have a computer and a Webcam.

Be a Volunteer

Cathy is a forty-three-year-old financial planner who is quite familiar with stress on the job. The main way she gets relief, she says, is by volunteering at the local no-kill animal shelter. After work two nights a week and for several hours on the weekends, Cathy visits, walks, and plays with dogs at the shelter and refers to them as her "children."

"I find myself looking at the clock on the days when I go to the shelter," she says. "The dogs are so much fun to be with, and they give unconditional love. Whenever I have some extra time during the week, I drive to the shelter and see how I can help out. I feel like they are my children, and whenever one is adopted, I feel a sense of loss while also feeling so glad one of my 'kids' has found someone to give them a home."

Cathy says a few of her family and friends have asked her why she wants to spend so much of her free time "working" with dogs and not get paid. "They don't understand how rewarding it is," she says. "I've tried to explain how the time I spend with the dogs is like going on vacation or a great playdate for me. I don't think about work or my problems. It's just me and the dogs and a few other volunteers who feel the same way, and it's great."

Cathy's sentiments about volunteering and experiencing great rewards in return are shared by millions of others who give of their time and energy. Whether you volunteer in a soup kitchen, read to children, clean up highways, hand out water during a marathon, visit the elderly in nursing homes, or clean dog runs, all are examples of altruistic acts. Being altruistic means you want to help people, animals, or the environment by doing good deeds without looking for personal gain, recognition, or rewards. However, as many volunteers like Cathy know, there can be tremendous personal rewards when you focus your energy and time on others, and much of that reward comes in the form of stress relief, better mood and perspective on life, and improved energy level.

When you volunteer your time and energy, it's important to have the right fit. If you strongly believe in the importance of reading and education, for example, you might find fulfillment in helping young children read or tutoring them in math skills. Or you may be an avid advocate of reading but not be fond of working with children, so helping adults who have difficulty reading might be a better fit for you.

An effective antidote for stress is helping others who are less fortunate than you. Most communities have programs run by churches, nonprofit organizations, hospitals, or schools that provide opportunities for people to volunteer their time to aid the homeless, individuals who are homebound, elderly people in need of companionship or assistance at home, veterans, abandoned or abused animals, or children. When you have an opportunity to focus on helping others who have problems, you can gain a better perspective on your own life and the things that are causing you stress and anxiety.

An interesting study published in *Gerontologist* in April 2012 reported on how early baby boomer women who were working anticipated volunteering during retirement. Although the study involved only nineteen women, the results were telling. The investigators found that the women indicated they would volunteer "for personal, not altruistic reasons, on their own terms through direct service; they are not interesting in the consuming commitments of board and committee work or fundraising," and that their volunteering "must be meaningful, something about which they are passionate and on their own schedule."

These women sound as if they know what they want. If they do, and if they follow through with their stated goals, then it is likely they will have fulfilling, stress-free or stress-reducing experiences as volunteers. Indeed, numerous studies have shown that volunteering is associated with an improved quality of life and social support. These benefits seem to be especially true for older adults, and most of the studies have focused on this age group, probably because retired people have more time to volunteer and also because of the health and socialization benefits associated with volunteering.

Some women have also discovered that spending time as a volunteer has improved their work and interpersonal relationships. Pauline, for example, has been married for thirty-five years and works part-time as a florist. She and her husband, Ralph, were in a rut. "Ralph is a management consultant, loves his job, and works long hours," she says. "He has work and golf buddies, and when he's home, we don't seem to have much to talk about anymore, now that the kids have moved away." Although she enjoyed her job, there wasn't much about it to discuss with Ralph. Pauline also was bored with the business party scene and found herself finding excuses to avoid the many social occasions Ralph had to attend. She felt she and Ralph were growing apart and that the lack of communication was putting a strain on their relationship.

Then Pauline decided to become a hospice volunteer for a local children's hospice. "I'm a firm believer in hospice, and the idea of hospice for children is something I wanted to explore," she says. After going through the training and beginning her work with patients, Pauline felt as if she had entered a whole new world, and she was eager to talk about it. "Suddenly I felt involved and excited," she explains. "Becoming a volunteer opened up communication with my husband and even socially. Ralph said to me, 'Wow, I haven't seen you this enthused about anything for years,' and he's right. Life seems more precious to me now, and so does my marriage."

ACTS OF KINDNESS

Performing random acts of kindness is, I believe, a wonderful way to banish stress and achieve a sense of calm and peace, even if these positive feelings last for only a short time. This belief has actually been backed up by research, but even if it were not, I'd still say that from personal experience, random acts of kindness are a valuable tool in the fight against stress—and this from a person who can be quite cynical. Here's an example.

Roselyn's Story

I met Roselyn while walking on the beach in winter in Delaware. It was the day after a big storm had moved through the area, and the sea had given up a wide range of shells and other objects not normally seen, so it was a beachcombers' delight, especially since the beach was mostly deserted. Roselyn and her dog, Chelsea, however, were braving the cold to look for shell treasures.

I had just discovered a particularly large conch shell, similar to one I had found the previous day during my walk on the beach. As I continued on my way, I saw Roselyn and her dog, and she was leaning over the sand, searching for shells. As I approached her, I asked if she had found anything interesting. She held up a small conch shell and said that's what she had found thus far.

When I showed her the shell I had found, she gasped and said how beautiful it was. I immediately offered it to her, saying I had found others yesterday and did not need to keep this one. I wanted her to have it. Again she was surprised and accepted the shell with much thanks.

It turned out we had much in common, and we talked for some time and made plans to get together again. And in fact, we did communicate via e-mail and met a few weeks later.

This chance encounter on the beach opened new possibilities for friendship, but perhaps more important, it was an affirmation that when we reach out to others with an open heart, something positive and uplifting can happen, even if the encounter lasts only a few minutes or less. When you make moments like this happen in your life, the focus is taken off the negative and the stress in your life is put aside, even if only briefly. However, you will still have the pleasant memory of the act of kindness and the way it made you feel.

Random acts of kindness may also relieve stress in the life of the receivers and even be the impetus for them to pass along their good feelings by performing random acts of kindness themselves. The encounter I had with Roselyn was not the first time I had participated in a random act of kindness with shells. More than a decade earlier, I was walking on the beach in Miami, worrying about a conference I had to attend later that morning. I discovered an especially beautiful shell and picked it up, slipping it into my pocket.

An elderly woman walking toward me was also searching for shells, and I remember feeling suddenly moved to give her my find. She was greatly surprised and asked me why I had given her the shell. "I'd like you to have it," I said, "but I'd also like you to give another shell that you find to someone else." She promised she would, and I walked on toward my conference. The memory of that day in Miami is still fresh in my mind, and it flashed again when I met Roselyn.

Would you like to try some random acts of kindness and see how they make you feel? Here are a few suggestions— and feel free to come up with lots of your own:

- Help an older person (or anyone who needs help) in the grocery store reach items on a shelf

- Pick up the tab for a stranger's breakfast, lunch, or dinner

- Let someone go in front of you in line at the store or bank

- Offer to rake the leaves, mow the lawn, or clean out the gutters for an elderly neighbor

- Write a thank-you letter (not an e-mail!) to someone who made a difference in your life

- Invite a lonely and/or elderly neighbor over for coffee

- Hold the door open for people

- Donate usable clothing, books, or other items to someone or an organization that can use them

- Help someone load or unload their groceries

- Smile and say good morning to the first ten people you meet each day

NATURE AND GETTING AWAY FROM IT ALL

Have you ever gotten away from all your worries and troubles and spent hours or days in nature, away from the stressful demands of work, cell phones, computers, and other hassles of a busy lifestyle? Taking such a step may be the most rewarding thing you ever do, and here's why.

Many people talk about how they feel less stress and anxiety when they "get away from it all" and spend time in nature, but few studies have actually documented these feelings. David Strayer, a University of Utah psychology professor, put it to the test and teamed up with two University of Kansas psychologists to study this phenomenon and eventually publish their findings in December 2012.

A total of fifty-six individuals (average age, twenty-eight years) of an Outward Bound expedition participated in the study. Twenty-four of the study participants took a ten-question creativity test before they left on the four- to six-day wilderness trip while the other thirty-four took the test on day four. Test results indicate that the participants scored 50 percent better on creativity after they had spent three nights in the wilderness, away from cell phones and computers.

What does this mean to you? According to author Richard Louv, who wrote *Last Child in the Woods: Saving Our Children from Nature-Deficit Disorder,* everyone wants to spend time in nature, but "we can't focus on it because of all of the distractions." In other words, the stress in your life prevents you from appreciating the wonders of nature. Does this sound familiar? Do you often feel the same way?

According to Louv, the need to connect with nature is critical. "We need that affiliation, that connection with nature. Without it, we do not remain fully human." Louv has called getting out in nature a dose of "vitamin N," noting that spending time in nature boosts our senses and can enhance our work productivity as well.

When was the last time you connected with nature

for at least a few hours and left your troubles behind? For many people, making that connection is an important part of their ability to cope with the stress in their lives. "Walking in the desert every morning has a way of lifting the stress from my shoulders," says one fifty-eight-year-old Tucson resident. "I can face the day better if I take that forty-five- to sixty-minute morning walk before work. I try to connect with or notice something new every time I take a walk, and when I think about that feature during the day, it makes me smile and I feel at peace."

While some people are blessed with easy access to natural surroundings, others are not. If getting out in nature is a challenge, here are a few suggestions:

- Seek out green places in your area: a small park, a nature sanctuary, even a greenhouse or nursery.

- If you have a backyard, create a garden with space for you to sit and be still. Be sure to include something that attracts birds, such as a feeder or birdbath.

- If you don't have a yard, create a small indoor garden with potted and hanging plants.

- Consider volunteering as a nature guide or mentor at a state park or nature park. Training is typically provided for these activities.

- Join a hiking or nature club or an environmental organization. These groups typically have events that will allow you to enjoy and learn more about nature.

BE AN ANIMAL'S BEST FRIEND

If you already are a pet parent to one or more dogs, cats, birds, or other creatures, then you already may be familiar with the joy and companionship they can bring. Dogs and cats are the most popular and common pets (companion animals) in the United States. According to the American Veterinary Medicine Association's publication, *U.S. Pet Ownership and Demographics Sourcebook* (2012), there are approximately 70 million pet dogs and 74.1 million pet cats in the United States. As of 2011, 63.2 percent of pet parents considered their pets to be family members.

Socializing with companion animals and other creatures can be one of the most rewarding and stress-reducing ways to spend your time. As an example, here's a study I like about women, stress, and dogs. All the women in the study had high-stress jobs (e.g., nurses, teachers, doctors, dentists, veterinarians). The women were asked to perform a difficult math task under one of three conditions: with the researcher in the room, with their best friend in the room, or with their dog in the room. Overall, the women responded as if threatened when they did the task in the presence of their best friend but as challenged when they were with their dog. In addition, the women who did the task with their dog in the room performed dramatically better than women who did the task with their friends or with the researcher.

But there's more to the story. Karen Allen, PhD, the study's lead author, explained that when she asked the women how they thought having a dog had an impact on their lives, all of them spoke of ways their dogs had assisted them during transitional times in their lives. Five of the women had become widows the year before the study, and what they all said is interesting, as Allen explains:

"Although their circumstances were somewhat different from each other, the descriptions they gave of the role of their dog in dealing with a husband's death were nearly identical. Each widow said that while she appreciated the consolation efforts of family and friends, she really wanted to be alone with her dog, especially immediately following her husband's death. Part of the reason was that the dog had been shared by the husband, but more important was the feeling that, with the dog, no social pretenses were necessary, and no one was judging her ability to 'bear up.'"

Other women who participated in the study also talked about how their dogs provided support during a divorce, when there were illnesses to deal with, and when they had problems at work with coworkers. Allen also noted that "a recurring theme was the use of imagery of the dog in times of high stress, and there were consistent reports that when the dog was imagined, obstacles appeared less daunting and difficult tasks more possible."

Benefits of Being a Pet Parent

If you already share your home with a pet, then you may want to think about the relationship you have with your companion and the benefits it brings. For example:

- Pet companions allow uncomplicated emotions. Relationships with people are complex, even in nonstressful situations, and when you are experiencing stress and anxiety, emotions can run high. That can lead to hurt feelings, getting advice (even if you don't want it), worrying about saying or doing the wrong thing, and dealing with a variety of personalities. Pets, however, are un-complicated. They listen without giving their opinion or advice, and they can be there for you without judgment.

- Pets can keep you active. One reason some peo-ple get a dog is to motivate them to get more physical exercise. Walking and playing with your dog can be effective stress reducers. If you walk your dog with a friend who also has a dog, then you are expanding your socialization op-portunities. While cats don't need to be walked, they do like to play (especially younger ones; older ones, not as much), and engaging in shared playtime activities every day is a great way to socialize with your kitty.

- Pets are companions. Feeling lonely, depressed, or neglected? If you have a companion animal, you have a friend who can help take the edge off feelings of loneliness, stress, or depression. If you live alone or come home to a house devoid of humans, what's better than being greeted by a wagging tail, a loving purr, and unconditional love?

- Pets can improve your health. Studies have shown that owning a dog or cat can lower your heart rate and blood pressure, reduce stress and anxiety, and elevate the good mood chemicals in the brain (see "Health Benefits of Having a Pet").

- Pets can improve self-esteem. Being a pet parent requires some level of responsibility, because it means you are charged with taking care of the health and well-being of the pet on a daily basis. Although shouldering this responsibility may be too much for some people, many find that caring for a dog or cat gives them a feeling of importance, self-satisfaction, and self-worth.

- Pets can help you socialize. What's one of the quickest ways to break the ice and strike up a conversation with a stranger? If that stranger is walking a dog, it's magnetic. Although many people would not even consider walking up to someone they don't know and initiating a conversation, a person with a dog on a leash is a magnet. If you are walking your dog as well or visiting a dog park, then socializing is practically guaranteed. Such situations are a win-win-win: the dogs have an opportunity to play, you get a chance to socialize, and a stress-reducing event takes place.

Health Benefits of Having a Pet

Scores of studies have examined the health benefits of being a pet owner/parent, and the advantages are especially evident in relation to stress and related factors such as anxiety, depression, and tension. Here are just a few of the findings:

- A Stanford University Medical Center study reviewed the literature on health and pet ownership and reported that people who have dogs are more physically active, have lower blood pressure and cholesterol levels, respond better to stress, and live longer after a heart attack than people who do not have a pet. The authors concluded that "overall, ownership of domestic pets, particularly dogs, is associated with positive health benefits."

• Remember the discussion about the "love hormone," oxytocin, in Step 1? Well, it's time to discuss it again, and this time the discussion concerns the relationship among pets, stress, and stress hormones, including oxytocin. A 2012 study in *Frontiers in Psychology* reported there is some evidence that interactions between people and animals reduces stress hormones such as epinephrine and norepinephrine, improves functioning of the immune system and the ability to manage pain, increases feelings of trust toward other people, reduces aggression, and improves learning. The authors also pointed out that oxytocin "plays a key role in the majority of these reported psychological and psychophysiological effects" of human-animal interactions. Therefore, it appears the benefits of interacting and socializing with pets is much more than emotional and superficially physical—it affects people at a cellular level.

• What kinds of biochemical activities occur when people and animals interact? A study published in *Veterinary Journal* looked at this question, and the results are eye-opening. The authors found that "concentrations of beta-endorphin, oxytocin, prolactin, beta-phenylethylamine, and dopamine increased in both species [people and dogs] after positive interspecies interaction." Another exciting finding was that levels of the stress hormone cortisol decline in people (but not in the dogs) after human-animal interaction. Thus it appears that people get much more benefit from human-companion animal interaction (or at least with dogs) than the animals do.

If you don't have a pet, there are ways you can enjoy the benefits of sharing time with a dog, cat, or other animals. For example:

- Contact a local animal shelter or rescue organization and ask about their fostering program. You may be able to foster a dog or cat until a home is found for the animal.

- Offer to walk and/or spend time with a pet that belongs to a family member, friend, or neighbor.

- Volunteer at a local animal shelter, zoo, or wildlife sanctuary. Many local, state, and federal organizations also offer programs where individuals can volunteer their time helping with a variety of animal welfare programs.

Although dogs and cats typically get the most attention when people talk about the benefits of pets for health and stress management, you can also experience stress relief by interacting with other animals. Watching fish in an aquarium can be very relaxing, and parakeets, canaries, parrots, and other birds can be excellent companions as well. Before becoming a parent to any animal, however, you should consider all the factors, including time you can spend with the animal, cost of care, your ability to care for the pet, and who can take care of the pet if you are unable to do so.

Pets and Stress at Work

If you're struggling with stress on the job, you might talk to your boss about bringing your dog to work with you. Although only about 20 percent of companies have policies that allow pets in the workplace, according to a 2009 survey conducted by the American Pet Products Association Manufacturers, the advantages for both employees and employers may cause that percentage to rise.

Some of those advantages were revealed in a 2012 study from Virginia Commonwealth University, in which investigators evaluated the impact of having dogs in the workplace at a manufacturing retail factory that employed about 550 people. The researchers collected saliva samples to measure stress hormone levels and also surveyed the employees, who were divided into three groups: pet parents who brought their dogs to work, pet parents who left their dogs at home, and people without dogs.

The investigators found that although levels of stress hormones did not change among the groups, the amount of stress people felt did. Specifically, employees who brought their dogs with them to work said they experienced less stress and more job satisfaction when compared with individuals who either did not bring their dogs to work or who did not have a dog. Overall, the employees were positive about the experience as well, especially in terms of stress relief and improved morale.

Among the other benefits of bringing dogs to the workplace are that pet parents do not need to worry about their pets being home alone all day and that the presence of the dogs can help to foster better relationships among coworkers.

"I work in a small office with about twenty people," says Clarissa. "When the boss began bringing her golden retriever, Molly, to work, the whole atmosphere in the office changed for the better. We saw the biggest change in our boss, who became more relaxed, which made everyone else feel more at ease and more cooperative and productive. I don't have a dog at home, but this experience has made me seriously consider adopting a companion for myself."

STEP 7

Bring in the Pros

IN THIS CHAPTER

Therapy and Stress
Religion, Spirituality, and Prayer
Emotional Freedom Technique
Medications for Stress

The Beatles told us all we need is love, but sometimes it takes a little more than love to defeat the ravages of stress. In chapter 2 I talked about how chronic stress can take a significant toll on your physical, emotional, mental, and spiritual health. When you suffer with headaches, recurring infections, stomach problems, and insomnia associated with stress, it's time to take action, and that may mean seeking professional help. If you dread getting up each morning and facing another day and there's little joy in your life, then stress is getting the best of you.

When stress takes over your life even though you've

tried DROP and various different ways to cope with or eliminate stressors and you're not getting relief—of even if you want some additional support—then it may be time to take the next step. Let's face it, everyone can use help once in a while, and even therapists seek solace from other therapists! Sometimes it takes an unbiased third party—someone who's not your mother or your best friend, partner, or sister—to shine a light into the dark corners of the psyche and to help identify hidden stressors or the most effective ways to cope with life's challenges.

That's where health professionals come in. Asking for help is not a sign of weakness. In fact, it takes great courage and strength to reach outside one's comfort zone. Brenda, a forty-eight-year-old freelance graphic artist, said she was literally "spinning around," not knowing which way to turn during a stressful time in her life, which finally prompted her to seek help.

"One night before dinner I was turning around in my kitchen, first one way and then the other. I felt so overwhelmed I couldn't even think straight to prepare dinner. All I wanted to do was cry. I had let the stress of trying to work at home while having my invalid mother move in with me take over my life. I was too paralyzed to take a rational, stress-reducing step on my own. I knew I needed help." Fortunately, Brenda found assistance from a counselor and group therapy, and also located respite from caring for her mother. Once she took that first step toward professional help, she began to feel some of the burden lifted from her shoulders and to feel more positive about her life.

Brenda was also fortunate she had not turned to dangerous and all-too-common means of coping with stress, such as excessive use of alcohol, illicit drug use, or misuse of prescription medications. She had, however, been experiencing sleep problems. Insomnia, along with weight loss and other physical side effects of chronic stress, frequently causes individuals to seek help from their physician, even though not all health-care professionals recognize and treat stress adequately (see chapter 2).

In this chapter I have expanded the definition of health professionals to go beyond doctors, therapists/counselors, psychologists, and psychiatrists to include spiritual advisors, who assist with healing the spirit. Included here are also discussions on the merits of cognitive behavioral therapy, EMDR (Eye Movement Desensitization and Reprocessing), group therapy, and medications.

HOW THERAPY HELPS STRESS

When was the last time you and your best friend—whether that friend is your sister, a coworker, someone you've known since grade school, or your partner—had your own therapy session? You know the kind I'm talking about: where you hash out a problem or challenging situation over coffee, a glass of wine, or during a brisk walk through the park? Such occasions are like informal therapy sessions.

But what about more formal counseling or therapy? Guidance from a mental health professional such as a counselor or therapist, psychologist, or psychiatrist may be the assistance you need to help move through your chronic stress and the impact it is taking on your body, emotions, and spirit.

There are several reasons why it can be beneficial to seek professional counseling. Although family and friends certainly can help women work through stressful times, sometimes people need a trained professional who can see and listen with a fresh, unbiased perspective.

Cognitive Behavioral Therapy

One type of formal therapy that has been shown to be effective in managing stress is cognitive behavioral therapy. The basic idea behind cognitive behavioral therapy for stress management is that life circumstances or events are not the cause of stress, but the way you perceive them is. Each person grows up learning and believing certain things and specific ways to perceive people and the environment. Cognitive behavioral therapy takes into account people's beliefs, perceptions, and influences in life and how they impact their reactions to stress.

Therapists who use cognitive behavioral therapy for stress management use talk therapy to influence negative feelings and emotions. The objective is to help individuals identify the association between the stress they experience and their irrational emotions and realize that negative feelings are counterproductive. As people begin to understand that their negative perceptions and beliefs are the cause of their stress, and that there are negative consequences to continuing with this way of thinking, they can then learn how to perceive circumstances and events in their lives in a more positive light.

Cognitive behavioral therapy is not a passive event, which is why it can be so effective for managing stress. Participants learn how to become more aware of their body and how it reacts to stress (e.g., muscle tension, heart rate, pain) and to reflect on those reactions. To reduce negative thinking, people are taught how to respond to situations, not react. This part of the therapy may involve writing down how you react to different problems so you can learn how to act in positive, constructive ways.

Another aspect of cognitive behavioral therapy is self-talk or internal dialogue, in which individuals learn to stop self-defeating thoughts and attitudes and restructure them into positive thinking and actions. Finally, therapists may encourage individuals to reflect or meditate on their goals, short-term and long-term, their quality of life, and on their relationships with others, as part of their overall plan to manage stress in their lives.

Finding Therapy Help

Counseling and therapy for stress management and related issues such as anxiety and depression are available through a variety of sources, including private practitioners, clinics, hospitals, universities, some employers, and religious/spiritual centers (whose leaders frequently have degrees in counseling). If you are not comfortable with or able to afford individual counseling, you can also inquire about group sessions.

You should also look for stress management lectures, workshops, and classes that are offered by any of the aforementioned individuals or facilities. Check out your local newspapers and Internet listings for such possibilities, and you also can contact individual hospitals, clinics, and similar facilities and inquire about any stress management options they offer.

RELIGION, SPIRITUALITY, AND PRAYER

Sometimes the most helpful and powerful forces in life are those that can't be physically held, measured, or seen. Religion, spirituality, and prayer are such forces for many people, who turn to God/higher power/higher energy, priests, ministers, shamans, gurus, or other spiritual leaders for guidance and help with stress, depression, anxiety, and other emotional turmoil in their lives.

The concept of spirituality means different things to

different people, but in general it involves a belief in a higher source or power that provides purpose or meaning to life, a set of values to live by, an acceptance that there are some things that are difficult or impossible to understand, and the concept that it's important to care about others. Religion shares many of the same concepts, but it tends to be more structured, possess dogma, and differ in emphasis, intent, and execution when compared with spirituality. One is not better or worse when it comes to being effective in managing stress and both, as is prayer, are highly personal.

According to Dr. Roberta Lee, author of *The Super Stress Solution*. "Research shows that people who are more religious or spiritual use their spirituality to cope with life," and that includes the ability to deal with stress. Such individuals also "heal faster from illness, and they experience increased benefits to their health and well-being," notes Lee. One reason for these advantages, says Lee, is that spirituality helps people connect with their world and thus allows them to "stop trying to control things" all by themselves. She explains that "when you feel part of a greater whole, it's easy to understand that you aren't responsible for everything that happens in life." That understanding is accompanied by relief from stress and anxiety.

The Power of Prayer and Religion

Prayer might be called the religious person's meditation, but perhaps the most important thing about prayer and meditation is that both can be effective in reducing stress, enhancing overall health, and relieving emotional unrest. Prayer and meditation also can be helpful if you are experiencing physical pain associated with stress.

Some people use prayer to help them cope with daily

frustrations and worries because it enables them to keep
the bigger picture in perspective. One such individual is
Sarah, whom I met during a trip to the Southwest. Sarah is
a bright, intense, thirty-something married woman who
was struggling to raise three children, one of whom has
cerebral palsy, largely on her own because her husband
was in Afghanistan most of the time as a civilian contrac-
tor. She lived in a small community in Idaho while her
parents and the rest of her family lived on the East Coast,
so she had no immediate family support. When I asked
her how she managed the stress in her life, her answer was
immediate.

"Prayer and my church," she said. "That's where I get
my strength. The minister at my church is very understanding and helpful, as are so many of the people in the
church. But when I'm alone and feel like it's all too much
for me, I pray and it gets me through."

Harold Koenig, MD, professor of psychiatry and behavioral sciences, and associate professor of medicine at
Duke University, as well as director of Duke University's
Center for Spirituality, Theology, and Health, evaluated
more than one thousand studies that explored the impact
of prayer and religion on health. He, along with his co-
authors, published their findings in the *Handbook of
Religion and Health*. In it they point out some intriguing
relationships between prayer, religion, and health. For
example:

- People with heart disease who do not practice religion are fourteen times more likely to die after
  undergoing surgery than individuals who practice religion.

- Individuals who say they are more religious tend
  to experience depression less than people who

are not religious, and they also tend to bounce back from their depression faster.

- Hospitalized patients who never go to church stay in the hospital an average of three times longer than people who go to services regularly.

Other studies have revealed more evidence that religion has a role in health and stress. For example, women who go to a religious service every week, regardless of their faith, may lower their risk of dying by 20 percent compared with women who don't go to services. Why? The authors of the study, which involved more than 92,000 women, aren't sure of the reason for the health benefit. Some possibilities, according to the study's head author, Eliezer Schnall, clinical assistant professor of psychology at Yeshiva College at Yeshiva University in New York City, are that attending services helps women feel a greater sense of community or less depressed, or they enjoy greater emotional and social support, which boosts their overall health.

These benefits have been noted elsewhere, and they make sense. Religion and attendance at any type of services provide an opportunity for socialization and support from church members, as well as a chance to offer support to others, all of which are elements that can reduce stress. Prayer and religion can provide some other stress-coping benefits as well:

- Religion offers structure in the form of dogma, commandments, expectations, and regulations, and this can give people a sense of stability and thus less stress. This does not mean everyone who says they follow a specific religion also adheres to its teachings, but people tend to identify with the religion because it gives them a sense of security and belonging.

• Religion can reinforce a belief system, which also provides a feeling of stability.

• Religion and prayer are associated with hope and purpose, and they can help provide people with the meaning of life. When life has meaning, uncertainty, stress, anxiety, and depression can be better managed.

In a 2012 French study subtitled "Does religion have a positive impact on mental health?" the authors explained that religion "might be a protective factor against several mental health problems." They noted that religions themselves likely are not the reason for this benefit, but that their components, such as "shared moral standards, social support, sense of meaning, purposefulness and control, and meditation habits, exercising an inhibiting influence on chronic stress," are the controlling factors.

At Georgia Southern University, a research team tackled an interesting question: What impact would a "supportive entity," God, have on acute stress? The investigators randomly assigned the student volunteers to one of three groups: prayer (reading a prayer), encouraging self-talk, and control. Then all the participants were exposed to a stressful situation. Overall, the participants in both the prayer and self-talk groups reported less stress than those in the control group. As further evidence, blood pressure levels among those who prayed were lower than among controls, although blood pressure levels were similar between people who prayed and those who engaged in self-talk. The authors suggested blood pressure levels were not more improved among those in the prayer group when compared with the self-talkers because most of the students did not consider reading a prayer to be the same as praying.

EMOTIONAL FREEDOM TECHNIQUE

If you haven't heard of Emotional Freedom Technique, or EFT, then you can now join the growing number of people who are trying and getting results from this stress-, fear-, and anxiety-reducing method. EFT is considered a self-help approach to stress management, and you can learn some basics on your own (see the appendix for information on EFT). However, since EFT combines cognitive therapy, exposure therapy, and acupressure, you may want to seek out the help of a professional. In addition, some people find that using EFT tapping on themselves is not as effective as when they do it along with a professional. That professional may be someone who has been trained in EFT only, or a doctor, nurse, psychologist, or other health-care professional who has added this healing method to their practice.

How EFT Works

Briefly, EFT has been described as a form of psychological energy medicine that is based on the same energy meridians used in acupuncture and acupressure. Instead of using needles or applying pressure to the points along these meridians, however, you use tapping with your fingertips on specific points on the chest and head while you focus on specific issues, such as the stress-causing situations in your life.

While tapping, you are supposed to voice positive affirmations, and the combining of these two activities is reported to help restore the body's bioenergy and relieve the emotional stress and other physical or emotional issues that have built up in your body and mind. An example of the general phrase used by those who practice EFT is: "Even though I have————, I deeply and completely accept myself." You fill in the blank with whatever stressful situation, negative emotion, or other issue you have in your life that you want to resolve.

For example, if you are experiencing stress over dealing with your teenagers, you might say, "Even though I have a problem dealing with my children, I deeply and completely accept myself." Advocates of EFT note that doing the tapping and repeating the affirmations in front of a mirror while staring in your eyes may strengthen the response, and that you should do the process up to ten times a day, especially before going to bed.

You might say, "But what if I don't believe the affirmation?" EFT practitioners emphasize that it doesn't matter whether you believe the affirmation; the important thing is to keep repeating it. Saying it out loud is best, although you can say it to yourself as well.

This is a simple explanation of EFT, and there are variations on the techniques used by different practitioners. If you are interested in learning more about EFT, see the appendix for resources.

Research on EFT

According to Dr. Gabor Mate, the author of *When the Body Says No: The Hidden Costs of Stress* and who uses EFT in his life for a variety of issues, EFT tapping can help people get their lives back on track. Dozens of controlled studies help support this claim.

Research into the impact of EFT for the management of stress, anxiety, phobias, depression, and other associated issues has been done with college and high school students, women with fibromyalgia, health-care workers, veterans, and others. One example of the effectiveness of EFT can be seen in the results of a study of more than one hundred health-care workers. All the individuals were assessed for emotional distress, pain, and cravings before and after they completed two hours of self-applied EFT during a workshop and then followed up ninety days later. Most of the participants used EFT after the workshop, and their assessment scores revealed the benefits. Significant improvements in distress, pain, and cravings were achieved, and the more the workers used EFT, the greater was their symptom relief.

Evidence that EFT can have an impact on cortisol levels was seen in a 2012 study in which eighty-three volunteers were randomly assigned to participate in an EFT group, a psychotherapy group that also involved supportive interviews, or no treatment at all. The researchers evaluated changes in cortisol levels and distress symptoms in all the participants before and after the interventions. Individuals in the EFT group showed significant improvements in anxiety, depression, and overall severity of symptoms when compared with the other two groups. In addition, cortisol levels in the EFT participants declined significantly when compared with those in the other two groups.

STRESS AND MEDICATION

Although many women find they can manage and cope with stress using a variety of nonpharmaceutical methods, sometimes it's necessary to get a little help from a medical doctor and her prescription pad. Abigail, a thirty-four-year-old mother of three-year-old twins who also runs an Internet business at home, felt as though she were falling apart from the combined stress of caring for her children and running the business.

"I was actually blessed because business was good, actually too good, and I couldn't handle it myself," she explains. "But at the same time, I didn't feel like I had the time or energy to find someone to help me and to train them while also caring for my kids, my husband—who travels a lot—and my house."

Abigail began losing sleep and suffering headaches. She resolved to practice deep breathing and try yoga, but her best intentions soon got pushed aside when her twins got the flu and she began having trouble with her computers. After experiencing two panic attacks within a few days of each other, she decided to call her doctor. He saw her and wrote a prescription for a low dose of fluoxetine, a type of antidepressant known as a serotonin reuptake inhibitor (see below) and encouraged her to talk to a therapist or counselor. Abigail did talk to her minister on several occasions, who urged her to try the deep breathing and yoga again.

After about a month of taking fluoxetine and doing the deep breathing, Abigail said she felt more balanced and much better able to handle the stress in her life. "I feel like the drugs took the edge off," she says, "and I felt more relaxed and capable of tackling and restructuring my life so I could better handle my work and my children. Then after another three months, I told my doctor I wanted to stop the drug."

During those few months, Abigail worked on establishing a better schedule using DROP—prioritizing her work each day, delegating certain tasks to her husband when he was home, maximizing and organizing her work space to optimize her workload and reduce stress. Eventually, she hired and trained someone to help her with her Internet business, and she feels more in control of her life.

Medications for Stress

If stress and anxiety have reached a point where it is difficult or impossible for you to conduct your daily activities and take care of yourself and your family, then you may need to talk to a medical professional about some short-term medication. Prescription drugs also can be helpful if you have experienced a traumatic event such as the death of a loved one or a major situation that has disrupted your life.

Physicians and psychiatrists (and psychologists in some states) can prescribe medications that cause sedative and tranquilizing effects. Those drugs typically are in the following categories and are associated with a variety of side effects. Before taking any type of medication, be sure to tell your health-care provider about any other medications, supplements, or other remedies you are using as well as any medical conditions you have.

- Barbiturates. This class of drugs is sometimes used for short-term relief of severe situational stress and anxiety. Drugs in this category include amobarbital (Amytal), butabarbital (Butisol), phenobarbital (Luminal), and secobartibal (Seconal). These drugs should not be used long term because they are associated with a high risk of physical dependency.

- Benzodiazepines. The drugs in this group are usually prescribed for long-term treatment of anxiety. Common drugs in this category include alprazolam (Xanax), chlordiazepoxide (Librium), clonazepam (Klonopin), diazepam (Valium), and lorazepam (Ativan). Long-term use of benzodiazepines can cause physical dependence.

- Buspirone. Although buspirone (Buspar) is an antianxiety drug, it is different from other drugs in this category. Physicians frequently prescribe buspirone for long-term treatment of generalized anxiety.

- Serotonin reuptake inhibitors (SRIs). Commonly prescribed drugs in this category include fluoxetine (Prozac), sertraline (Zoloft), and paroxetine (Paxil). These medications are often used long term to treat anxiety disorders, stress, and panic disorders.

- Serotonin-norepinephrine reuptake inhibitors (SNRIs). This group is the latest among antidepressants. SNRIs are prescribed for severe stress, anxiety, social anxiety, and panic disorders. Drugs frequently prescribed in this group include duloxetine (Cymbalta) and mirtazapine (Remeron).

All of these drugs are associated with significant side effects, which can include dry mouth, nausea, vomiting, rash, blurry vision, urinary problems, swallowing problems, dizziness, fatigue, shortness of breath, wheezing, mouth ulcers, and other symptoms. In addition, the Food and Drug Administration (FDA) requires that the makers of SRIs and SNRIs include a special black box warning on their products concerning an increased risk of suicidal thoughts or behaviors in individuals who use these drugs, especially children, adolescents, and young adults, within the first few weeks of use.

If you turn to professionals for help with stress management, be sure to let them know about any other nutritional or herbal supplements, drugs, or treatment approaches you are using or have used in the past and your results, as they may have an impact on your treatment results and what they choose to suggest.

ENDNOTES

Chapter 1

Kreider T. The busy trap. *New York Times,* June 30, 2012. Accessed Nov. 26, 2012: http://opinionator.blogs.nytimes.com/2012/06/30/the-busy-trap/

Marin M-F et al. There is no news like bad news: women are more remembering and stress reactive after reading real negative news than men. *PLoS ONE* 2012. DOI:10.1371/journal.pone.0047189

Ornish D et al. Increased telomerase activity and comprehensive lifestyle changes: a pilot study. *Lancet Oncology* 2008 Nov; 9(11): 1048–57

Taylor SE et al. Biobehavioral responses to stress in females: tend-and-befriend, not fight-or-flight. *Psychology Review* 2000 Jul; 107(3): 411–29

WebMD. Why men and women handle stress differently. http://women.webmd.com/features/stress-women-men-cope?page=2

Chapter 2

Ahola K et al. Work-related exhaustion and telomere length: a population-based study. *PLoS ONE* 2012 Jul; 7(7): e40186. DOI: 10.1371/journal.pone.0040186

Almeida D et al. Penn State University. Accessed Nov. 3, 2012: http://live.psu.edu/story/62452

Bermudez-Rattoni F, ed. *Neural Plasticity and Memory: From Genes to Brain Imaging.* Boca Raton: CRC Press, 2007.

Beth Israel Deaconess Medical Center study. Accessed Nov. 22, 2012: http://www.medicalnewstoday.com/releases/252999.php

Cohen S et al. A global measure of perceived stress. *Journal of Health and Social Behavior* 1984; 24: 386–96

Epel ES et al. Accelerated telomere shortening in response to life stress. *Proceedings of the National Academy of Science USA* 2004; 101(49): 1732–25

Homann D et al. Stress perception and depressive symptoms: functionality and impact on the quality of life of women with fibromyalgia. *Rev Bras Reumatol* 2012 May–Jun; 52(3): 319–30

Leuner B. Mood disorders: Animal models of stress and depression. October 13, 2012, at the annual meeting of the Society for Neuroscience in New Orleans. http://www.eurekalert.org/pub releases/2012-10/osu-csd101012.php

National Heart Lung and Blood Institute. Accessed Dec. 21, 2012 http://www.nhlbi.nih.gov/health/health-topics /topics/hdw/

Norberg M et al. Work stress and low emotional support is associated with increased risk of future type 2 diabetes in women. *Diabetes Research in Clinical Practice.* 2007 Jun; 76(3): 368–77

Perricone, Nicholas. *The Wrinkle Cure: Unlock the Power of Cosmeceuticals for Supple, Youthful Skin.* New York: Warner Books, 2000.

Pervanidou P, Chrousos GP. Metabolic consequences of stress during childhood and adolescence. *Metabolism* 2012 May; 61(5): 611–19

Pouwer F et al. Does emotional stress cause type 2 diabetes mellitus? A review from the European Depression in Diabetes (EDID) Research Consortium. *Discovery Medicine* 2010 Feb: 9(45): 112–18

Richardson S et al. Meta-analysis of perceived stress and its association with incident coronary heart disease. *American Journal of Cardiology* 2012 Dec 15; 110(12): 1711–16

Volkow, Nora D. in Thea Singer's *Stress Less.* New York: Hudson Stress Press, 2010, p. 100

Step 1

American Massage Therapy Association: Accessed Nov. 10, 2012: http://www.amtamassage.Org/articles/2 /PressRelease/detail/2545

Balk J et al. The relationship between perceived stress, acupuncture, and pregnancy rates among IVF patients: a pilot study. *Complementary Therapies in Clinical Practice* 2010 Aug; 16(3): 154–57

Cuneo CL et al. The effect of Reiki on work-related stress of the registered nurse. *Journal of Holistic Nursing* 2011 Mar: 29(1): 33–43

Denner SS. The science of energy therapies and contemplative practice. A conceptual review and the application of Zero Balancing. *Holistic Nursing Practice* 2009 Dec; 23(6): 315–24

Duncan AD et al. Employee use and perceived benefit of a complementary and alternative medicine wellness clinic at a major military hospital: evaluation of a pilot program. *Journal of Alternative and Complementary Medicine* 2011 Sep; 17(8): 809–15

Dias M et al. Effects of electroacupuncture on stress-related symptoms in medical students: a randomised controlled pilot study. *Acupuncture in Medicine* 2012 Jun; 30(2): 89–95

Edmonds D, and G. Gafner. Touching trauma: combining hypnotic ego strengthening and zero balancing. *Contemporary Hypnosis* 2003; 20(4): 215–20.

Engen DJ et al. Feasibility and effect of chair massage offered to nurses during work hours on stress-related symptoms: a pilot study. *Complementary Therapies in Clinical Practice* 2012 Nov; 18(4): 212–15

Fixler M et al. Patient experience of acupuncture provision in a GP practice. *Complementary Therapies in Clinical Practice* 2012 Aug; 18(3): 140–44

Kober A et al. Auricular acupressure as a treatment for anxiety in prehospital transport settings. *Anesthesiology* 2003 Jun; 98(6): 1328–32

Lindgren L et al. Physiological responses to touch massage in healthy volunteers. *Autonomic Neuroscience* 2010 Dec 8; 158(1–2): 105–10

Listing M et al. The efficacy of classical massage on stress perception and cortisol following primary treatment of breast cancer. *Archives of Women's Mental Health* 2010 Apr; 13(2): 165–73

Moyer CA et al. Does massage therapy reduce cortisol? A comprehensive quantitative review. *Journal of Bodywork and Movement Therapy* 2011 Jan; 15(1): 3–14

Toms R. Reiki therapy: a nursing intervention for critical care. *Critical Care Nursing* 2011 Jul–Sep; 34(3): 213–17

Wentworth LJ et al. Massage therapy reduces tension, anxiety, and pain in patients awaiting invasive cardiovascular procedures. *Progressive Cardiovascular Nursing* 2009 Dec: 24(4): 155–61

Step 2

Complete Guide to the Alexander Technique: http://alexandertechnique.com/

Kemper K et al. Nurses' experiences, expectations, and preferences for mind-body practices to reduce stress. *BMC Complementary and Alternative Medicine* 2011 Apr 11; 11:26

Kuramoto AM. Therapeutic benefits of tai chi exercise: research review. *WMJ* 2006 Oct; 105(7): 42–46

Puterman E et al. The power of exercise: buffering the effect of chronic stress on telomere length. *PLoS One* 2010 May 26; 5(5): e109837

Wang WC et al. The effect of tai chi on psychosocial well-being: a systematic review of randomized controlled trials. *Journal of Acupuncture and Meridian Studies* 2009 Sep; 2(3): 171–81

Watson, Rita. Activity, Sex, Laughter and Meditation are Stress Relief Secrets. *Psychology Today* 2012 Jul. 16. Accessed online Nov. 25, 2012. http://www.psychologytoday.com/blog/love-and-gratitude/201207/activity-sex-laughter-and-meditation-are-stress-relief-secrets-237

Wolever RQ et al. Effective and viable mind-body stress reduction in the workplace: a randomized controlled trial. *Journal of Occupational Health Psychology* 2012 Apr; 17(2): 246–58

Yadav RK et al. Efficacy of a short-term yoga-based lifestyle intervention in reducing stress and inflammation: preliminary results. *Journal of Alternative and Complementary Medicine* 2012 Jul: 18(7): 662–67

Step 3

Aselton P. Sources of stress and coping in American college students who have been diagnosed with depression. *Journal of Child and Adolescent Psychiatric Nursing* 2012 Aug; 25(3): 119–23

Ball, Jeanne. Women and stress: why we meditate. Accessed Nov. 2012. http://www.huffingtonpost.com/ jeanne-ball/women-and-stress-why-we-m_b_944023 .html

Berk LS et al. Neuroendocrine and stress hormone changes during mirthful laughter. *American Journal of Medical Science* 1989 Dec; 298(6): 390–96.

Hayama Y, Inoue T. The effects of deep breathing on "tension-anxiety" and fatigue in cancer patients undergoing adjuvant chemotherapy. *Complementary Therapies in Clinical Practice* 2012 May; 18(2): 94–98

Interview with Goldie Hawn in *Prevention* magazine, accessed Nov. 30, 2012, at http://omg.yahoo.com/news /healthy-hollywood-fab-food-friday-goldies-anti-aging -163943863.html

Karagozoglu S et al. Effects of music therapy and guided visual imagery on chemotherapy-induced anxiety and nausea-vomiting. *Journal of Clinical Nursing* 2012 Nov 8

Kashani M et al. Novel stress reduction technique improves sleep and fatigue. Chest 2012; 142(4): 1052A. doi: 10.1378/chest. 1361738

Marc I et al. Mind-body interventions during pregnancy for preventing or treating women's anxiety. *Cochrane Database of Systematic Reviews* 2011 Jul 6; (7): CD007559

Miller M, and WF Fry. The effect of mirthful laughter on the human cardiovascular system. *Medical Hypotheses* 2009 Nov; 73(5): 636–39

Murray MT, and JE Pizzarno. Stress management. In Pizzorno JE, Murray MT, eds. *Textbook of Natural Medicine* 3rd ed, 2006. Vol 1, pp. 701–8. St. Louis: Churchill Livingstone.

Rogers KR et al. Guided visualization interventions on perceived stress, dyadic satisfaction and psychological symptoms in highly stressed couples. *Complementary Therapy in Clinical Practice* 2012 May; 18(2): 106–13

Step 4

Amen DG, MD, brain imaging specialist. Cravings and brain addiction. Article retrieved Dec. 10, 2012: http://www.newsmaxhealth.com/dr_amen/cravings_brain_addiction/2010/08/03/338093.html

Chen WW et al. Pharmacological studies on the anxiolytic effect of standardized schisandra lignans extract on restraint-stressed mice. *Phytomedicine* 2011 Oct 15; 18(13): 1144–47

Conrad P, and C. Adams. The effects of clinical aromatherapy for anxiety and depression in the high risk postpartum woman—a pilot study. *Complementary Therapies in Clinical Practice* 2012 Aug; 18(3): 164–68

Dang H et al. Antidepressant effects of ginseng total saponins in the forced swimming test and chronic mild stress models of depression. *Progress in Neuropsychopharmacology Biology Psychiatry* 2009 Nov 13; 33(8): 1417–24

Edwards D et al. Therapeutic effects and safety of Rhodiola rosea extract WS1375 in subjects with life-stress symptoms—results of an open-label study. *Phytotherapy Research* 2012 Aug; 26(8): 1220–25

Fortuna JL. Sweet preference, sugar addiction, and the familial history of alcohol dependence: shared neural pathways and genes. *Journal of Psychoactive Drugs* 2010 Jun: 42(2): 147–51

Hongratanaworakit T. Aroma-therapeutic effects of massage blended essential oils on humans. *Natural Product Communications* 2011 Aug; 6(8): 1199–204

Kennedy DO et al. Modulation of cognition and mood following administration of single doses of ginkgo biloba, ginseng, and a ginkgo/ginseng combination to healthy young adults. *Physiology Behavior* 2002 Apr 15; 75(5): 739–51

Lee S et al. Schizandra chinensis and Scutellaria baicalensis counter stress behaviors in mice. *Phytotherapy Research* 2007 Dec; 21(12): 1187–92

Olsson EM et al. A randomised, double-blind, placebo-controlled, parallel-group study of the standardised extract shr05 of the roots of rhodiola rosea in the treatment of subjects with stress-related fatigue. *Planta Medica* 2009 Feb; 75(2): 105–12

Reay JL et al. Panax ginseng (G115) improves aspects of working memory performance and subjective ratings of calmness in healthy young adults. *Human Psychopharmacology* 2010 Aug; 25(6): 462–71

Srivastava JK et al. Chamomile: a herbal medicine of the past with bright future. *Molecular Medicine Reports* 2010 Nov 1; 3(6): 895–901

University of Maryland Medical Center; accessed Dec. 20, 2012: http://www.umm.edu/altrned/articles /aromatherapy-000347.htm#ixzz2Fc1e1bus

Wesnes KA et al. The memory enhancing effects of a Ginkgo biloba/Panax ginseng combination in healthy middle-aged volunteers. *Psychopharmacology (Berl)* 2000 Nov; 152(4): 353–61

Step 5

Bungay H, Clift S. Arts on prescription: a review of practice in the U.K. *Perspective in Public Health* 2010 Nov; 130(6): 277–81

Leckey J. The therapeutic effectiveness of creative activities on mental well-being: a systematic review of the literature. *Journal of Psychiatric and Mental Health Nursing* 2011 Aug; 18(6): 501–9

Pinniger R et al. Argentine tango dance compared to mindfulness meditation and a waiting-list control: a randomized trial for treating depression. *Complementary Therapies in Medicine* 2012 Dec; 20(6): 377–84

Tango dancing can ease stress, anxiety and depression. *Prevention:* http://www.prevention.com/mind-body /emotional-health/tango-dancing-can-ease-stress-anxiety -depression#ixzz2GBmmu9d8

Toyoshima K et al. Piano playing reduces stress more than other creative art activities. *International Journal of Music Education* 2011 Aug; 29: 3257–63

Turiano NA et al. Openness to experience and mortality in men: analysis of traits and facets. *Journal of Aging & Health* 2012 Jun: 24(4): 654–72

Step 6

Allen K at al. Presence of human friends and pet dogs as moderators of autonomic responses to stress in women. *Journal of Personality and Social Psychology* 1991; 61: 682–89.

Allen K. Coping with Life Changes & Transitions: The Role of the Pet. Online at Pet Partners (formerly DeltaSociety), accessed Dec. 30, 2012: http://www .petpartners.orq/document.doc?id=113

Arhant-Sudhir K et al. Pet ownership and cardiovascular risk reduction: supporting evidence, conflicting data and underlying mechanisms. *Clinical and Experimental Pharmacology & Physiology* 2011 Nov; 38(11): 734–38

Atchley RA et al. Creativity in the wild: improving creative reasoning through immersion in natural settings. *PLoS ONE* 2012: 7(12): e51474

Barker RT et al. Preliminary investigation of employee's dog presence on stress and organizational perceptions. *International Journal of Workplace Health Management* 2012; 5(1): 4. Online: http://www.emeraldinsight.com /journals.htm?articleid=17024849&show=abstract

Beetz A et al. Psychosocial and psychophysiological effects of human-animal interactions: the possible role of oxytocin. *Frontiers in Psychology* 2012; 3:234

Mills H et al. Socialization and altruistic acts as stress relief. Updated June 30, 2008. At MentalHelp.net

Morrow-Howell N et al. Who benefits from volunteering? Variations in perceived benefits. *Gerontologist* 2009 Feb; 49(1): 91–102

Odendaal JS, Meinties RA. Neurophysiological correlates of affiliative behavior between humans and dogs. *Veterinary Journal* 2003 May; 165(3): 295–301

Parkinson L et al. Volunteering and older women: psychosocial and health predictors of participation. *Aging & Mental Health* 2010 Nov; 14(8): 917–27

Peters S et al. Differential effects of baclofen and oxytocin on the increased ethanol consumption following chronic psychosocial stress in mice. *Addiction Biology* 2012 Nov 6.

Prettyman B. Put down the iPhone and take a hike: your creativity will soar, Utah researcher says. *Salt Lake Tribune* 2012 Dec. 12. Accessed Dec. 12, 2012. http:// www.sltrib.com/sltrib/news/55444364-78/nature-louv -strayer-technology.html.csp

Seaman PM. Time for my life now: early Boomer women's anticipation of volunteering in retirement. *Gerontologist* 2012 Apr; 52(2): 245–54

USA Today. Dogs allowed: creature comforts at the workplace. February 25, 2009: http://usatoday30.usatoday .com/life/lifestyle/2009-02-24-pets-office N.htm

Watson, Rita. Activity, Sex, Laughter and Meditation are Stress Relief Secrets. *Psychology Today* 2012 Jul. 16. Accessed online Nov. 25, 2012. http://www.psycologytoday .com/blog/love-and-gratitude/201207/activity-sex-laughter -and-meditation-are-stress-relief-secrets

Step 7

Belding JN et al. Social buffering by God: prayer and measures of stress. *Journal of Religion and Health* 2010 Jun; 49(2): 179–87

Brattberg G. Self-administered EFT (Emotional Freedom Techniques) in individuals with fibromyalgia: a randomized trial. *Integrative Medicine: A Clinician's Journal* 2008 Aug-Sep; 30–35

Church D, Brooks AJ. The effect of a brief EFT (Emotional Freedom Techniques) self-intervention on anxiety, depression, pain and cravings in healthcare workers. *Integrative Medicine: A Clinician's Journal* 2010 Oct-Nov; 40–44.

Church D et al. The effect of emotional freedom techniques on stress biochemistry: a randomized controlled trial. *Journal of Nervous and Mental Disease* 2012 Oct; 200 (10): 891–96

Koenig H et al. *Handbook of Religion and Health.* 2nd ed. New York: Oxford University Press, 2012.

Korneich C, Aubin HJ. Religion and brain functioning (part 2): does religion have a positive impact on mental health? *Revue Médicale de Bruxelles* 2012 Mar-Apr; 33(2): 87–96

Schnall E et al. The relationship between religion and cardiovascular outcomes and all-cause mortality in the Women's Health Initiative Observational Study. *Psychology & Health* 2010 Feb; 25(2): 249–63

APPENDIX

SUGGESTED READING

Basil, Casie, and Center for Healing Through Aromatherapy. *Healing through. Aromatherapy: Your 2-Week Guide to Taming Your Stress, Calming Your Mind and Healing Your Body.* Spartus Group LLC, 2012.

Branch, Rhena, and Rob Willson. *Cognitive Behavioural Therapy Workbook for Dummies.* West Sussex, England: John Wiley & Sons, 2007.

Brennan, Richard. *The Alexander Technique Workbook: The Complete Guide to Health, Poise and Fitness,* London: Collins & Brown, 2011.

Brown, Kristen K. *The Happy Hour Effect: Twelve Secrets to Minimize Stress and Maximize Life.* Norwood, NJ: Goodman Beck Publishing, 2012.

Brown, Richard, and Patricia Gerbarg. *The Healing Power of the Breath: Simple Techniques to Reduce*

Stress and Anxiety, Enhance Concentration, and Balance Your Emotions. Boston MA: Shambhala Publications, 2012.

Carlson, Richard. *Don't Sweat the Small Stuff . . . and It's All Small Stuff.* New York: Hyperion, 1996.

Davis, Martha, et al. *The Relaxation and Stress Reduction Workbook.* Oakland, CA: New Harbinger Publications, 2008.

Desy, Phylameana I. *The Everything Guide to Reiki: Channel Your Positive Energy to Promote Healing, Reduce Stress, and Enhance Your Quality of Life.* Avon MA: Adams Media 2010.

Dossey, Larry. *Prayer Is Good Medicine: How to Reap the Healing Benefits of Prayer.* New York: Harper Collins, 1996.

Dossey, Larry. *Healing Words: The Power of Prayer and the Practice of Medicine.* San Francisco: HarperCollins, 1993.

Editors of Reader's Digest. *Massage and Aromatherapy: Simple Techniques to Use at Home to Relieve Stress, Promote Health, and Feel Great.* New York: Reader's Digest, 2011.

Gach, MR, and Beth Ann Henning. *Acupressure for Emotional Healing: A Self-Care Guide for Trauma, Stress, and Common Emotional Imbalances.* New York: Bantam, 2004.

Gawain, Shakti. *Creative Visualization: Use the Power*

of Your Imagination to Create What You Want in Your Life. Novato, CA: New World Library, 2002.

Hanson, Rick. *Stress-Proof Your Brain: Meditations to Rewire Neural Pathways for Stress Relief and Unconditional Happiness.* Sounds true Inc., 2010.

Jones, Frank Pierce. *Freedom to Change—The Development and Science of the Alexander Technique.* Mouritz, 1997.

Lawlis, Frank. *Retraining the Brain: A 45-Day Plan to Conquer Stress and Anxiety.* New York: Penguin, 2009.

Lawrence, Grade. *Stress Relief Foods and Recipes.* CreateSpace Independent Publishing Platform, 2012.

Malchiodi. Cathy A. *Art Therapy Sourcebook.* New York: McGraw Hill, 2006.

Marsi, Martin. *Power Vibrancy Massage Guide: How to Unleash Your Super Human Potential and Eliminate Stress with a 10-Minute Self-Massage System.* Martin Marsi Communications, Kindle Edition, 2012.

McClellan, Stephanie, and Beth Hamilton. *So Stressed: The Ultimate Stress-Relief Plan for Women.* New York: Free Press, 2010.

Moss, Charles A, and Peter Eckman. *Power of the Five Elements: The Chinese Medicine Path to Healthy Aging and Stress Resistance.* Berkeley, CA: North Atlantic Books, 2010.

NurrieSterns, and Rick NurrieSterns. *Yoga for Anxiety:*

Meditations and Practices for Calming the Body and Mind. Oakland, CA: New Harbinger Publications, 2010.

Perricone, Nicholas. *The Wrinkle Cure: Unlock the Power of Cosmeceuticals for Supple, Youthful Skin*. New York: Warner Books, 2000.

Pickhardt, Carl E. *Stop the Screaming: How to Turn Angry Conflict with Your Child into Positive Communication*. New York: Palgrave Macmillan, 2009.

Prasad B, Grandhi P. *The Turning Point: Conquering Stress with Courage, Clarity and Confidence*. Cedar Fort, Inc., 2012.

Quest, Penelope. *Reiki for Life: The Complete Guide to Reiki Practice for Levels 1, 2 and 3*. New York: Penguin, 2010.

Reinhardt, Annie, and Viktor Reinhardt. *The Magic of Touch: Healing Effects of Animal Touch and Animal Presence*. Washington, DC: Animal Welfare Institute, 2010.

Rones, Ramel, and David Silver. *Sunset Tai Chi: Simplified Tai Chi for Relaxation and Longevity*. Wolfeboro, NH: Ymaa Publication Center, 2011.

Seaward, Brian Luke. *Managing Stress: Principles and Strategies for Health, and Well-Being*. Burlington MA: Jones & Bartlett Learning, 2011.

Singer, Thea. *Stress Less: The New Science That Shows Women How to Rejuvenate the Body and the Mind*. New York: Hudson Street Press, 2010.

Stahl, Bob, et al. *A Mindfulness-Based Stress Reduction Workbook*. Oakland CA: New Harbinger, 2010.

Talbott, Shawn, and William Kraemer. *The Cortisol Connection. Why Stress Makes You Fat and Ruins Your Health—and What You Can Do About It*. Alameda, CA: Hunter House, 2007.

Vredevelt, Pam, and Jean Lush. *Women and Stress*. Grand Rapids, MI: Revell, 2011.

Winston, David, and Steven Maimes. *Adaptogens: Herbs for Strength, Stamina, and Stress Relief*. Rochester, VT: Healing Arts Press, 2007.

Benagh, Barbara, and Michael Wohl. *Yoga for Stress Relief*. DVD, 2006.

WEB SITE RESOURCES

All Things Healing

A comprehensive Web site that is an "online community for healing mind, body, spirit, planet," and is chock-full of articles and useful information on everything from acupressure and massage to energy medicine, herbalism, holistic nutrition, and the human /animal bond.
http://www.allthingshealing.com/

American Psychological Association

Stress reduction tips
http://www.apa.org/helpcenter/stress-tips.aspx

Alexander Technique

A complete guide to the Alexander Technique
http://alexandertechnique.com/

Apps for Stress Reduction

There are dozens—perhaps scores—of apps you can get
to help with stress reduction. Just insert the words "apps
for stress" into your favorite search engine and you'll
come up with lots of Web sites from which you can get
free or very low-cost apps.

Care Pages

CarePages Web sites are patient blogs that are free and
allow individuals to connect with their family and
friends during a health challenge. Can be helpful for
women who are going through stressful times and who
need some social support.
https://www.carepages.com/

Daily Strength

A Web site that offers a vast network of support groups
ranging from anxiety and depression to obesity, financial
worries, and panic attacks.
http://www.dailystrength.org/

Emotional Freedom Technique

Complete information about EFT, including free
instructions, help locating practitioners, research on
EFT, and a list of upcoming workshops.
http://www.eftuniverse.com/

Guided Visualizations

Inner Health Studio offers a wide range of visualization scripts online for stress management.
http://www.innerhealthstudio.com/visualization-scripts.html

Healthy Place

This Web site says it is the "largest consumer mental health site," and it offers information on psychological disorders and psychiatric drugs, as well as has a social network for support, online psychological tests, videos, and more. Healthy Place offers information on anxiety, depression, insomnia, and other issues associated with chronic stress.
http://www.healthyplace.com/

Homeopathic Pharmacopoaie of the United States

In-depth information about homeopathy and homeopathic remedies.
http://www.hpus.com/overview.php

International Center for Reiki Training

Learn all you want to know about Reiki and its benefits, how to find practitioners, and more.
http://www.reiki.org/faq/whatisreiki.html

National Association for Cognitive Behavioral Therapists

This Web site offers not only information and research on cognitive behavioral therapy, but also a schedule of webinars on the topic.
http://www.nacbt.org/whatiscbt.htm

Pet Partners (formerly Delta Society)

Information and benefits about the animal-human bond.
http://www.petpartners.org/page.aspx?pid=333

Strictly Stress Management

Information and videos about art therapy for stress
management.
http://www.strictly-stress-management.com/art-therapy
-activities.html

Zero Balancing

Information about Zero Balancing and where to find
practitioners.
http://www.zerobalancing.com/